Power,
Politics,
and Policy
in Nursing

Rita Reis Wieczorek, R.N., Ed.D., F.A.A.N., is the Assistant Director of Nursing for the Clinical Career Pathway at The Mount Sinai Medical Center in New York City. For the past 20 years, she has taught Maternal-Child Nursing and Research to undergraduate and graduate students in various colleges and universities in New York City and San Antonio, Texas. Dr. Wieczorek received her undergraduate degree in nursing at the College of Mount Saint Joseph on the Ohio, her master's degree in nursing at New York University, and her doctorate in education at Teachers College, Columbia University. Dr. Wieczorek has co-authored a pediatric textbook, and published many articles and chapters in books primarily in the fields of nursing research, pediatric nursing, and nursing service management. She is a fellow in the American Academy of Nursing, and a member of several honor societies, while also serving on the board of directors of several associations and organizations. Dr. Wieczorek is the editor of the District 13 newspaper and serves as a referee to several journals of nursing. She is currently a Director at Large, the New York State Nurses Association.

POWER, POLITICS, AND POLICY IN NURSING

Rita Reis Wieczorek, R.N., Ed.D., F.A.A.N.,
Editor

SPRINGER PUBLISHING COMPANY
New York

Springer Publishing Company, Inc.
200 Park Avenue South
New York, New York 10003

85 86 87 88 89 / 10 9 8 7 6 5 4 3 2 1

Library of Congress Cataloging in Publication Data

Main entry under title:

Power, politics, and policy in nursing.
   This book is an outgrowth of the Nineteenth Annual Stewart Conference on Research
in Nursing held April 23, 1982, at Teachers College, Columbia University; sponsored
by the Nursing Education Alumni Association in Cooperation with the Dept. of Nurs-
ing Education at Teachers College.
   Includes bibliographies and index.
   1. Nursing—Political aspects—United States—Congresses. 2. Nursing—Social as-
pects—United States—Congresses. 3. Medical policy—United States—Congresses. I.
Wieczorek, Rita Reis. II. Stewart Conference on Research in Nursing (19th : 1982 : Teachers
College, Columbia University) III. Columbia University. Nursing Education Alumni
Association. IV. Columbia University. Teachers College. Dept. of Nursing Education.
[DNLM: 1. Delivery of Health Care—United States—congresses. 2. Health Policy—
United States—congresses. 3. Nursing—trends—United States—congresses. 4. Politics
—United States—congresses. W3 ST313 19th 1982p / WY 16 P8875 1982]
RT86.5.P69 1984   362.1'73'0973   84-13931
ISBN 0-8261-4630-9

Printed in the United States of America

Contents

Preface

There has been little written or researched on the topics of power, politics, and policy in the nursing literature. Perhaps nurses and others do not think of the nursing role as one that has power, effects health policy, and is active in the political scene on the local, state, and national levels. Nursing has been struggling with its professional identity and image for years. These struggles can be traced from the Nightingale era to contemporary society. Over the years, progress has been made and standards of practice have been raised, both of which are reflected in the improved educational background of nurses, the expanded practice of nurses in a technological world, advances in areas of health maintenance and prevention, and the development of a larger leadership core as more persons in nursing assume executive positions in the health care industry, education, and government.

Nurses need to focus on and deal with the theme of this book. Nurses want power in their places of employment. Power should be based on the level of knowledge, skill, experience, and area of responsibility. A few nurses are impacting on governmental health policy. Some nurses are becoming active in the political/legislative arenas. Nurses must be involved in legislation related to nurse practice acts, health care reimbursement policies, and laws or regulations that affect the health of the society which they are privileged to serve.

Power, Politics, and Policy was the theme of the Nineteenth Annual Stewart Conference on Research in Nursing held April 23, 1982, at Teachers College, Columbia University. This book is an outgrowth of that conference.

Over the past 20 years, the Nursing Education Alumni Association, in cooperation with the Department of Nursing Education at Teachers College, has sponsored an annual research conference to share with other nursing scholars current research studies primarily completed by alumni from their graduate programs. The studies were usually unpublished doctoral dissertations completed within the past five years. In

1982, Rita Reis Wieczorek was selected chairperson of the Stewart Research Conference. She directed a committee composed of 14 alumni members and a faculty representative from the Department of Nursing Education, Teachers College. Over 300 persons attended the research conference.

As the Stewart Conference was being planned, changes in the format were decided. The theme—*Power, Politics, and Policy*—was chosen first, then both doctoral and postdoctoral research studies were evaluated for presentation. Researchers invited to participate in the conference were directed to address the conference theme in their work. Respondents to the studies were chosen on the basis of their knowledge and expertise in research on the topic and their ability to critique the study in relationship to the conference theme. Researchers were asked to focus on the findings and implications of their investigations. Lengthy presentations of sampling techniques and statistical analysis were avoided.

The five studies included in this book have also been presented at the Stewart research conferences. Four were selected from the 1982 program and one was selected from the 1981 program. (All studies in the book focus on concepts of power, politics, and policy that are significant to nursing in the 1980s and 1990s.)

The 19 essays selected for this book were contributed by members of the Committee of the Conference on Research in Nursing, by keynote speakers, panel presenters at the Stewart Conference, as well as some other nurse leaders in the country. The editor solicited works on as broad a range of topics as deemed appropriate for the purposes of this book.

The contributors include nurse researchers, educators, deans, and directors from undergraduate, graduate, and doctoral nursing programs, nurse practice executives, nurse organizational executives, nurse business executives, nurse governmental executives, and nursing service executives.

The views expressed in the book are solely those of the contributors. In editing the book, no attempt was made to change the ideas or thoughts expressed by the contributors. In fact, the editor believes that one of the most exciting things in this book is the personal analysis of the topics by the contributors. They do vary in their opinions of the concepts of power, politics, and policy in nursing. The ideas and research in the book span a continuum from nursing as a profession which has no power, no political clout, and little input into policy, to the all-knowing, all-powerful, politically astute and policy-making health professional group. Perhaps nursing fits on a point somewhere between these two extremes on the continuum.

The purpose of this book is not to determine if the nursing profession has made "good, fair, or bad marks" in the arenas of power, politics, and policy but it is to generate in the reader a commitment to the development of the profession through the use of these concepts. This book gives the reader an idea of where the profession has come from, where it is now, and what its hopes are for the future. It does not matter if you completely agree with the viewpoints, experiences, and research presented by the contributors; the important thing is to read the book and make your own plan to gain power, use politics, and establish policy where you study and work. The point is to live your life more effectively through power, politics, and policy.

Acknowledgments

I would like to thank some of the people who helped me accomplish the task of producing a contemporary book on power, politics, and policy in nursing by nurses. They were: my family—Robert, Bob, and Randa; Carole Saltz, director of the nursing program at Springer whom I met in Hawaii at an American Nurses Association Convention about 10 years ago; and Amy Friedman, a brand new writer friend who types in between ''real jobs'' such as writing movies and novels; thank you all very much. Your support was appreciated. Writers need discipline and all of you provided the structure that enabled me to share with others the contributed works in *Power, Politics, and Policy in Nursing*.

Contributors

Myrtle K. Aydelotte, Ph.D., R.N., F.A.A.N., is currently a nursing consultant, Adjunct Professor at the University of Iowa College of Nursing, and Clinical Professor at Yale University. She received her baccalaureate in nursing education at the University of Minnesota, where she also earned her Ph.D. She is a member of Sigma Theta Tau, a fellow of the American Academy of Nursing, and a member of the Institute of Medicine, National Academy of Science.

Elaine E. Beletz, Ed.D., R.N., F.A.A.N., is Associate Professor for Nursing at Villanova University College of Nursing with primary assignment for teaching nursing administration in the graduate program. She is the past president of the New York State Nurses Association and is a current member of the board of directors of the American Nurses Association, and the board of trustees of Nurses Coalition for Action in Politics. Dr. Beletz is a fellow of the American Academy of Nursing and a member of Sigma Theta Tau nursing honor society.

Patricia Westbrook Blagman, Ed.D., R.N., is an Associate Professor of Nursing, The Lienhard School of Nursing, Generic Masters Program, Pace University, Pleasantville, New York. She received a diploma in nursing from Presbyterian Hospital, New York City. She earned a B.S., M.Ed., and Ed.D. from Teachers College, Columbia University. She is a member of the American Nurses Association and Sigma Theta Tau. She has taught decision making in baccalaureate and higher degree programs for a number of years.

Vernice Ferguson, M.A., R.N., F.A.A.N., is Deputy Assistant Chief Medical Director for Nursing Programs and Director of Nursing Service for the Veterans Administration in Central Office, Washington, D.C. She is a fellow of the American Academy of Nursing and has served as its president. She is president-elect of Sigma Theta Tau, nursing's honor society; following a 2-year term she will become president. She is a faculty member in the schools of nursing at Georgetown University and the University of Maryland.

Keville C. Frederickson, Ed.D., R.N., is a Professor and the Associate Dean for Faculty and Academic Affairs at Pace University, The Lienhard School of Nursing. She received her B.S. from Columbia University School of Nursing and her M.Ed. and Ed.D. from Teachers College, Columbia University. She has been on the faculty at Columbia University School of Nursing and New York University, Division of Nursing, where she was Director, Center for Continuing Education in Nursing.

Ann Costello Galligan, Ed.D., R.N., is an Associate Professor in the Department of Nursing at the College of Mount Saint Vincent, Riverdale, New York. She received a B.S. in nursing from Boston College, an M.S.N. from Boston University, and an Ed.D. from Teachers College, Columbia University. Presently, she is a trainee in family therapy at the Center for Family Learning in New Rochelle, New York. Dr. Galligan is a member of Sigma Theta Tau as well as various professional organizations.

Valentina Harrell, Ph.D., R.N., is a clinical psychologist in private practice in New York City and a nurse educator who holds a joint appointment at Teachers College, Columbia University, in the Departments of Psychology and Nursing Education. She teaches courses in psychosocial aspects of health and illness, and nursing research and theory. She earned her bachelor of science in nursing and master of science degrees at Ohio State University, and is coauthor of *The Promotion of Physical Comfort and Safety*.

Lucille A. Joel, Ed.D., R.N., F.A.A.N., is Professor and Director for Clinical Affairs at Rutgers College of Nursing in New Jersey. In addition, she is Director of the Rutgers Teaching Nursing Home Project, which is one of 11 national sites funded by the Robert Wood Johnson Foundation to unify the efforts of nursing education and service. Dr. Joel received a B.S.N. from Seton Hall University in New Jersey, and continued at Teachers College, Columbia University, where she earned an M.A., an M.Ed., and an Ed.D.

Patricia Anne Jones, M.S.N., R.N., is the chief executive officer of Professional Nurse Associates, Inc., a Washington, D.C.-based health policy and program consulting firm. Ms. Jones holds expertise in health care financing, reimbursement systems, and professional review programs. Most recently, Ms. Jones served as Director of the American Nurses Association's Washington Office and Center for Governmental Affairs, where she was responsible for the implementation of the association's public policy, government relations, and political action programs. Ms. Jones' graduate degree is from the Catholic University of America.

Helen M. Lerner, Ed.D., R.N., is Assistant Professor and Coordinator of Parent-Child Nursing at Herbert H. Lehman College of The City University of New York. She received her B.S. in nursing from Skidmore College and her master's and doctor's degrees from Teachers College, Columbia University. She is a member of many professional organizations and has a number of publications and presentations on the subjects of nursing education, parenting, and developmental disabilities.

Marion D. Lewis, Ed.D., R.N., is Chairperson and Director of the Upper-Division Baccalaureate Nursing program at the State University College at New Paltz. She received the B.S.N. from Case Western Reserve University, the M.S. in psychiatric mental health nursing from Hunter College, and the M.Ed. and Ed.D. in higher education administration from Teachers College, Columbia University. Prior to her present position, Dr. Lewis was Associate Professor and Director of the undergraduate program, School of Nursing, State University of New York at Stony Brook.

Pamela Maraldo, Ph.D., R.N., is Executive Director of the National League for Nursing (NLN). She holds a bachelor of science in nursing degree from Adelphi University, New York, and a master's degree in nursing and doctor of philosophy degree from New York University. In her former position as Director of NLN's Office of Public Affairs, she managed preparation and presentation of testimony on health policy. She has published articles and presented numerous speeches on health policy issues, and has conducted survey research on related topics.

Margaret L. McClure, Ed.D., R.N., F.A.A.N., is the Executive Director of Nursing at New York University Medical Center; she is also an Adjunct Professor of Nursing at New York University. She is a fellow in the American Academy of Nursing, a member of Sigma Theta Tau, and currently president-elect of the American Society for Nursing Service Administrators. She is an active consultant and has published widely in the area of nursing administration.

Diane O'Neill McGivern, Ph.D., R.N., F.A.A.N., is an Associate Professor and Associate Dean at the University of Pennsylvania in Philadelphia. She graduated from St. John College in 1961 with a bachelor of science in nursing. The clinical focus of her graduate work was adult health and illness, and she received her Ph.D. in nursing from New York University, Division of Nursing, in 1972. Her areas of specialization are care of the adult, primary care, and curriculum development.

Erline P. McGriff, Ed.D., R.N., F.A.A.N., is a Professor in the Division of Nursing, School of Education, Health, Nursing and Arts Professions at New York University, where she was formerly head of the Division of Nursing from 1975 to 1982. She is a graduate of the Lucy Webb Hayes School of Nursing, Sibley Memorial Hospital in Washington, D.C.; she received the B.S. and M.S. from the Catholic University of America, and the Ed.D. from Teachers College, Columbia University.

Patricia Ruth Mixon, Ed.D., R.N., is presently an Assistant Professor in the graduate program, School of Nursing, Wright State University. She earned a diploma in nursing from St. Mary's School of Nursing, Huntington, West Virginia, a B.S.N. from Florida State University, and an M.Ed. and Ed.D. from Teachers College, Columbia University. She is a member of the American Nurses Association, National League for Nursing, Midwest Nursing Research Society, Society for Research in Nursing Education, Zeta Phi, and Sigma Theta Tau.

Lois G. Muzio, M.Ed., R.N., is a Mentor in Health Sciences at Empire State College, State University of New York, and a doctoral candidate at Teachers College, Columbia University. She received a diploma in nursing from Roosevelt Hospital School of Nursing in New York City and her B.S.N. and M.Ed. from Teachers College, Columbia University. She is a member of the American Nurses Association and the National League for Nursing. Her interests are adult education and adult development.

Janet N. Natapoff, Ed.D., R.N., is Professor and Director of Curriculum and Research at The City College School of Nursing in New York City. She received her B.S. from Alfred University, her M.S. from Boston University, and her Ed.D. from Teachers College, Columbia University. She is a member of several professional organizations, including the American Nurses Association, Sigma Theta Tau, and the Council of Nurse Researchers. For several years she has been involved in nursing legislative activities in New York State.

Andrea B. O'Connor, Ed.D., R.N., is Associate Professor of Nursing Education and Director, Center for Nursing Leadership Development, Teachers College, Columbia University. She holds a B.S.N. from Cornell University–New York Hospital School of Nursing, an M.A. from New York University, and an Ed.D. from Columbia University. Her present area of research involves the continuing education needs and patterns of participation of graduate-prepared nurses holding positions of authority and influence in educational and service settings.

Joan G. O'Leary, Ed.D., R.N., is an Associate Professor in the Graduate Program in Nursing Service Administration at Villanova University, College of Nursing. She is also President of O'Leary and Associates, Inc., a nursing management consulting firm that specializes in developing support systems for nursing service administrators. These systems include computerized nursing information systems, as well as management support systems for diagnostic-related groups.

Franklin A. Shaffer, Ed.D., R.N., is Deputy Director for Operations at the National League for Nursing (NLN). In this position he is responsible for direction and management of all NLN member programs and the initiation of new products and services. On the staff of the League since 1981, Dr. Shaffer has directed the NLN Forum for Nursing Administrators and continuing education programs nationwide for nurse managers. He initiated development of the NLN Council of Nursing Service for Hospitals and Related Facilities and the League's Nurse Executive Placement Service.

Elizabeth Dorsey Smith, Ed.D., R.N., F.A.A.N., is the Assistant Director of Nursing, Maternal-Child Health Division, at The Mount Sinai Medical Center in New York City. She has served previously as an Associate Professor, both at Hunter College in the School of Nursing and the Women's Studies Program and at Cornell University School of Nursing. She received her undergraduate degree at Duke University and completed her graduate work at Teachers College, Columbia University.

Barbara J. Stevens, Ph.D., R.N., F.A.A.N., is Director of the Division of Health Services, Sciences and Education at Teachers College, Columbia University. She also is the Chairman of the Department of Nursing Education and holds the Isabel Maitland Stewart Professorship of Nursing Education. She received her A.D. in Nursing from St. Petersburg Junior College, St. Petersburg, Florida; her B.S. from Northwestern

University, Evanston, Illinois; her M.A. from DePaul University, Chicago; and her Ph.D. from the University of Chicago.

Christiana Gomboschi Wasserman, M.Ed., R.N., is presently Assistant Director of the Center for Nursing Leadership and Administrative Associate to the Division Director, Division of Health Services, Sciences and Education, Teachers College, Columbia University. She has held positions in clinical practice, education, and nursing service administration, and has served as marketing consultant to professional and educational organizations. She is currently completing doctoral studies in nursing service administration at Teachers College, Columbia University.

Cathryne A. Welch, Ed.D., R.N., is Executive Director of the New York State Nurses Association. She is a graduate of the School of Nursing of the Robert Packer Hospital, Sayre, Pennsylvania, and earned bachelor of science, master of arts, and doctor of education degrees from Teachers College, Columbia University. Dr. Welch has had extensive involvement in revision of the laws defining and governing nursing practice in New York State and in diverse organizational activities related to nursing economics, education, practice, and services.

Margret S. Wolf, Ed.D., R.N., is the Director of the Advanced Education in Nursing Science Program in the Division of Nursing at New York University. She holds the bachelor in nursing degree from Hunter College of the City University of New York, and an M.Ed. and Ed.D. from Teachers College, Columbia University. Dr. Wolf is the coauthor of *Simulation/Games in Nursing Education,* and she is the author or coauthor of numerous articles and monographs relating to treatment environments, group behavior, and the development of simulations/games for the teaching of nursing.

Part I

ESSAYS

The first section of this book consists of 19 essays written by nurse leaders on the topics of power, politics, and policy in nursing, the "Three P's" which are crucial in any profession. The essays were subdivided into six central themes. Clearly, many of the ideas discussed overlap with one another, and some essays could be included easily in more than one of the six sections. The subdivisions were created primarily to present an organized flow of information to the reader. Our intention was to incorporate varied points of view as well as different approaches to the analysis of a concept related to one or more of the three P's. The themes in order of presentation in Part I are: an overview of the concepts of power, politics, and policy; governmental perspectives; power in nursing; nursing education; roles of professional nursing associations; and professional change and marketing. The contributors' essays represent their own viewpoints, based on their professional, educational, and workplace experiences. The 19 essays in Part I tell us where nursing is in the 1980s; some brave contributors have made suggestions for change in the 1990s.

The first two essays were contributed by Ferguson and Stevens, respectively. Ferguson lists three models—power, education, and organization—that can be useful for the analysis of the concepts in this book. She also outlined three views for the future. Perhaps the most interesting of these is one that lists seven traits said to be necessary for our descendants. Stevens begins with a description of new political behaviors in the workplace. She describes politics as "the domain of practical decision making." Stevens describes for readers the political climate of regulation for the baccalaureate degree as entry into professional nursing. This type of legislation is before the executive bodies of many states. Stevens ends her essay with a discussion of policy formulation and nursing. Basically she thinks, as others do, that nursing needs to initiate major health policy, not simply react to the health policies proposed by others.

Three essays address the theme entitled Governmental Perspectives. Shaffer's essay is related to Public Law (PL) 98–21 which focuses on prospective reimbursement policies for hospitals. The prospective payment policy is based on the new ''buzz word'' in the health care industry, diagnostic-related groups (DRGs). The new payment system began on October 1, 1983. There were five states exempted from the initiation date. In DRGs, patients upon discharge from the hospital are placed into the 467 diagnostic groups based on the following diagnoses: age, treatment procedure, discharge status, and sex. Shaffer overviews the impact he projects this new policy will have on the nursing profession. He is concerned that hospitals will seek cheaper labor in lieu of registered nurses. Shaffer thinks the nurse is in a pivotal position to make the new health care reimbursement work in the hospital setting. This could be done by viewing nursing as a revenue-producing cost center. Power in nursing can be exercised if one regards the system of the nurse monitoring the patient in the hospital as an efficient, cost-effective method of caring for patients. Good nursing care should lead to a shorter hospital stay for patients, which, in turn, leads to a greater cost-effectiveness than there would be if lower levels of personnel were responsible for delivering patient care services. Because DRGs are important to nursing power, policy, and politics, Shaffer's essay is the longest in Part I. He did his doctoral dissertation in this area and has been recognized as one of the leaders in nursing related to this topic. Jones' essay focuses on the effect of Reaganomics on the health care system and how it affects nursing. She worked in Washington, D.C. in the American Nurses' Association office when the essay was written. Jones gives the reader a first-hand governmental perspective on power, politics, and policy at the national level and how this impacts on nursing. The last essay related to this theme was contributed by McGivern. She discusses for the reader her experiences as a Robert Wood Johnson Health Policy Fellow in 1981–1982 in Washington, D.C. McGivern's assignment was to work with Senator Durenberger. He was chairman of the Health Subcommittee of the Senate Finance Committee. This Committee was responsible for financially managing the Medicare and Medicaid entitlement programs. At the time of McGivern's assignment, the Committee was considering the issue of federalizing Medicaid. Politics, power, and health policy were experienced first-hand by the contributor. She was responsible for interpreting health care needs to a governmental committee from the perspective of nursing.

The theme—power in nursing—is discussed in the next section in terms of conflicts and dilemmas. There are a total of six contributed essays which cover the following issues: feminism and nursing; how much power nursing does or does not have in the health care system; the amount and type of nursing research on power; how to obtain and use power; the perception of power is power; power and approaches to change; how political scientists view power and its relationship to nursing; group theories and how they affect power in nursing; and the developmental needs of nursing in relationship to power behavior. This general theme has more contributors than any other, probably because nursing has had more gains in the power arena than in politics and policy. The editor thinks that in the late 1980s and early 1990s, there will be a focus in nursing on using political strategies to initiate health policy by nursing on all levels of government.

McClure's essay was presented to the reader first in this section because it contains definitions and an overview of the power construct. It also addresses the fact that there have been few in-depth nursing studies done on power. Maraldo does a marvelous job demonstrating how the perception of power is power. As the new executive director of the National League for Nursing who comes from a background of political activity in nursing, she presents to the reader expertise on where nursing has been in power and politics and where it is going. This essay presents strategies that can be used by nurses to achieve more power in their work environment and in the government. In the words of Maraldo, "Power is the art of impression management." Smith presents two essays that address this theme: one focuses on competition and cooperative approaches, and the other focuses on career versus job orientation. Both of these essays relate feminism to the profession of nursing. Smith has some interesting viewpoints about women and nursing, how women treat other women in the profession, and what effects the women's movement has had on the nursing profession. Wolf's essay deals with power in nursing from a group theories perspective. She discusses sources of power and the group process in nursing. This is a rather different perspective than the other contributors have chosen in their essays. The editor believes that Wolf's essay derives from her development and research in psychiatric and mental health nursing. Developmental concepts are used by Harrell in her essay on power. She compares the development of power in nursing to the principles of growth and development. Harrell's mastery is an example of success and power.

The fourth theme is concerned with nursing education and its relationship to power, politics, and policy. There were three contributors that addressed this topic. Lerner's essay focused on the development of power in nursing education. She described several issues involved in socializing nursing students to see themselves as persons with power. These issues were: the image of professional nursing; the education of students to recognize the value in the autonomous function of nursing; and the realization that knowledge and skill is power. Muzio's essay, on the other hand, deals with politics in nursing education based on her personal experiences. In this essay, she describes the political in-group in education as being made up of those programs that promote the traditional type of nursing baccalaureate programs; she describes the political out-group as being made up of those programs that encourage alternate approaches to nursing education. Muzio's analysis of the Regents' External Degree Program and the proposed Empire State College Program in New York State provides the reader with a "bird's-eye-view" of internal politics in education. The tone of the essay is less than positive. Galligan's essay discusses women in nursing and how they have been socialized to view power and independence as negative characteristics. She believes that the nursing profession has been slow to internalize the feminist's underlying message of self-determination and commitment. Galligan's vision of nurses who perceive themselves as victims in the health care industry should be modified as women develop power during their periods of basic education.

The fifth theme is the role of professional nursing associations in the development of power, politics, and policy. Joel and Welch have contributed essays related to this section in Part I. Joel's essay addresses power through the professional association, and Welch addresses policy. These persons are experts in the area of professional associations, and they represent the leadership in our country in the 1980s.

The last theme is focused on professional change and marketing of the profession. The editor placed three essays in this section because she saw them all related to power, politics, and policy in the 1990s. Aydelotte's essay on professional change gives the reader direction and strategies for implementation of nursing power and policy. Beletz focuses on trade unions and nurses' rights. Wasserman's essay is directed to marketing the profession to the consumer and the larger society. This is an area about which nursing has a lot to learn and in which it must make strides to implement needed improvements.

Part I presents the essays on the topics of power, politics, and policy. Research studies are contained in Part II. With each research study is a response to that study. The five nursing research studies are a combination of doctoral and post-doctoral investigations.

Overview of the Concepts of Power, Politics, and Policy in Nursing

Power, Politics, and Policy in Nursing

Vernice Ferguson

INTRODUCTION

Power, politics, and policy are timely topics for discussion in the nursing profession. It is these three areas of influence that will determine the direction of nursing education, research, and practice in the 1980s and the 1990s. The time has now come for nurses to act powerfully and politically to influence and formulate health policy. The health care system in the United States needs to become more effective and at the same time focus on cost containment in the delivery of health care services. The federal, state, and local governments are demanding that these changes take place as soon as possible. Consumers are vocal in their demand for and evaluation of health services.

Nursing care can and must play a leadership role in the changes needed in the health care system. This can be accomplished by the use of power and politics in establishing, changing, and implementing needed health policy changes over the next two decades.

The Work Force and Potential Power Base

Who are the nurses? What are the characteristics of the climate in which they practice? What trends are evident? What does the future hold?

First, who are the nurses? For the second time in four years, a very rich data source is available. It is *The Registered Nurse Population, An Overview* (DHHS, 1980), from the national sample survey of registered nurses. The earlier one was conducted in 1977 and was summarized by Moses and Roth (1979). Out of 1.4 million nurses who held an active license to practice as a registered nurse, 17,000 participated in the study sample in 1977. There were 978,234 nurses actively employed in nursing, 68 percent on a full-time basis. The majority—an estimated 600,000 nurses—were employed in hospitals. This marked an increase of 16 percent over 1972 (Moses & Roth, 1979).

This time around, with 30,000 nurses surveyed, the 1980 data estimates that there are 1.6 million registered nurses in the United States who hold current licenses to practice. Approximately 76 percent of them—1.2 million nurses—are employed in nursing. Once again, the majority of nurses—more than 810,000—are employed in hospitals. Nearly 99,000 nurses work in nursing homes and extended care facilities, an increase in numbers over the last survey data. It is also notable that the majority of employed nurses have titles that reflect staff nurse positions. Another 57,000 are in specialty positions predominantly geared toward direct patient care, which is the major activity of most nurses who practice (DHHS, 1980).

Reputations are made, enhanced, and lost in the hospital environment. Cooley (1902) reminds us that "the imaginations people have of one another are the solid facts of society" (p. 10). Consider the power potential of those who practice in hospitals. Leaders in nursing need to determine whether what they do as they engage in their work affects this group in a significant way. Will those who practice in hospitals, primarily as staff nurses, join their leaders as they posture on behalf of nursing and nurses? Is there a common bond that is compelling enough to receive the attention of both groups? Does the hospital nurse who practices at two a.m. in the hospital, for example, know that what their leaders do and say makes a difference as she or he practices? Does the consistent outcome of the nurse's effort establish nursing as a credible and essential profession?

ASSESSMENT OF THE ENVIRONMENT

J. E. Anderson (1975) addressed the policy makers and their environment. In his view, systems theory suggests that policy making must be considered within the context of the environment in which it takes place. While the environment limits and constrains what policy makers accomplish, it becomes clear that the demands for policy actions are generated in the environment and transmitted to the political system. The environment includes geographical characteristics and demographic variables such as population size, age distribution, gender dominance, and spatial location as well as social, political, economic, professional structure and relationships. Other nations become a significant part of the environment as foreign, domestic, defense, political, and economic policies are formulated and implementation strategies developed. The larger order influences the direction of a nation, its programs, priorities, and the allocation of resources.

Witness, for example, the goals, objectives, and direction of the federal government. The dominant themes in the new federalism have become a strong national defense effort and a diminished role of the federal government in social welfare programs and the promulgation of regulations. The "buzz" words suggesting a change in direction are entitlement, volunteerism, self-reliance, individual, family, and private sector initiatives and responsibility. Do more with less remains the challenge.

Nurses need to learn to use marketing techniques and information as they expand their power base to influence politics and policy formulation. Commercial marketing experts are already responding to their surveys of population trends. Presently, the west and southwest account for more than half of all consumers. Despite the nation's slower population growth during the 1970s, southern and western markets grew much faster than expected. The population shift, west of the Mississippi and south of the Mason-Dixon line, will influence the marketing of consumer goods and services. Consider, for example, the current fashion of prairie-style skirts and silver-toned, western-styled jewelry as well as home decor.

It is expected that southern and western lifestyles will influence, in a major way, the development of new products and services. New laws will reflect increasingly the concerns of these high population growth areas as well. We can look to the people west of the Mississippi and south of the Mason-Dixon line to influence national policy issues as well. Is nursing preparing for this opportunity to influence the shape and direction of health care services? Is nursing formulating a definitive position as health care goals for people are planned and realized?

Newspaper headlines and captions tell a story too. Some reflect the effects of a constrained economy, while others present demographic variables which become significant as the future is planned. Some of the headlines and captions follow:

FRUSTRATED STUDENTS REALIZING THEY MUST
LOWER EXPECTATIONS
Job-Seekers Reassess Career Possibilities

COLLEGE STUDENTS AT PEAK, U.S. FINDS
Data List 12.3 Million On Rolls This Fall

WOMEN HEADED FAMILIES

U.S. CHILDREN OF THE 1980s;
MOST HAVE MOTHERS IN THE WORK FORCE

REPORT SHOWS 4 AMERICANS IN 10 ARE UNDER 25

SHARP RISE OF ELDERLY POPULATION IN '70s
PORTENDS FUTURE INCREASES

PARENTS DEMANDING PARTNERSHIP IN CHILD CARE

WORK FORCE IN '70s BETTER EDUCATED
(Selected newspaper headlines and captions, *The New York Times*
and *The Washington Post*, 1981, 1982).

Broad societal trends drive policy formulation. Three major forces continue to shape the real world. Nurses must respond to them as nursing is practiced in this arena where power, politics, and policy prevail. These forces are (1) a change in lifestyle; (2) a change in family relationships; and (3) a change in the status of women. The Urban Institute's three-year research program on women and family policy is another major contribution to the earlier ones in housing, health, and employment (Smith, 1979). Since nursing is a profession comprised predominantly of women, these findings are of significance as nursing's position in the arenas of power, politics, and policy are addressed.

Who will work in the future? By 1990, 52 million women will be working or looking for work, 11 million more than in 1978. Most will be married and many will have young children. Approximately 3.1 million are expected to be in the labor force with children under age six (Smith, 1979). The need for child care facilities is apparent. The implications for health care teaching present new opportunities. Entrepreneurial ventures for nurses in a new market can become creative initiatives for those who seek challenges. The seeking of political office on a responsive campaign platform can capture votes for nurses and other previously unknown candidates.

What kinds of work do women do? The institute's findings showed that one-third of the women engage in clerical work, while one-fourth are employed in health care (not including physicians), education (not including higher education), domestic service, and food service. Labor force participation for all women approximates 50.8 percent, while for nurses it is 76 percent (Smith, 1979). Nurse power in the marketplace does not match nurse participation in the labor force. Strategies are required to bolster participation which is in synchrony with labor force representation. Overcrowding is the biggest problem facing women in the labor market today, hence depressed salaries and higher unemployment. The vigorous pursuit of achieving equity through the Doctrine of Comparable Worth (meaning payment for work equals work actually done) is a rational one.

POWER

Who needs power? Nurses do. Why? Nurses must be able to get things done on behalf of the people nurses serve. Nurses serve clients who are consumers of nursing services. It is imperative that nurses learn and utilize the helping model, well known in rehabilitation and mental health nursing practice. Four features are readily evident: (1) the client and professional are active; (2) a trusting relationship develops over time; (3) problem solving, including successes and failures, is evident; (4) future problems can be handled by the client as a result of the helping relationship (Anderson, T. P., 1975).

Nurses must develop constituents. Nurses need to hold open house for consumers; nurses need to plan conferences with and for consumers. Nurse educators and nurse administrators need to make course content in schools of nursing and activities in service settings of interest and applicable to students of other disciplines.

The dimensions of power require understanding and skilled application. Power is gained, maintained, expanded, shared, and even given up. Determining the suitable dimension requires consensus development among nurses concerning the critical issues. Nursing's power base is constrained as long as nurses fail to reach agreement on the educational base required for the practice of nursing and the credential(s) denoting its achievement.

Nursing's power base can be expanded as nurses encourage and support nurse candidates for political office. Consider the political acumen and sophistication that nurse leaders develop with the professional association, other professional organizations, educational institutions, and service organizations. Nurses must marshal this tremendous potential as political office is pursued in an organized and united way.

Governance, management, and the performance of program activities enable institutions to achieve results through the organized efforts of people. Figure 1.1 depicts this relationship as a power model. Nursing as a profession is comprised predominantly of women. Women comprise the majority of today's college population, as well as the student population in this nation's business schools. Yet, as society achieves its work, few women are evident in the governance arena, a larger number perform as managers once policies have been formulated in the governance arena, while the majority are engaged in carrying out the program activities as work is accomplished without significant input in policy making. A strategic planning process is required to achieve a deserved place for nurses as the power model is reapportioned.

Knowledge is power. It confers upon the possessor authority. The initial preparation for nursing and the continued learning required to practice professionally must be systematic and substantive. This preparation is not easy to acquire nor sustain considering all that must be learned to assure a credible practice by competent nurses. Figure 1.2 portrays an educational model which prescribes three areas for core learning required of all nurses, human relations core, scientific-technical core, and organization core. The position which the nurse holds and the role performed determine the dominant core in which the greatest knowledge and skill are required.

POLITICS

J. Alexander McMahon, president of the American Hospital Association, once defined politics as substance and procedure, the art of living together and the "dirty" part, the interplay of power and expediency (Anderson, J. E., 1975).

Nurses are the largest number of health care professionals. Politically, however, nurses as influentials are acknowledged primarily at a time of crisis and compromised all too often at other times. Consider the hospital in which the majority of this nation's nurses practice—more than 810,000 of them. Figure 1.3 is a service organizational model with a hospital orientation in which the principle dyad that provides direct care to patients is the physician and the nurse. The nurse's versatility and

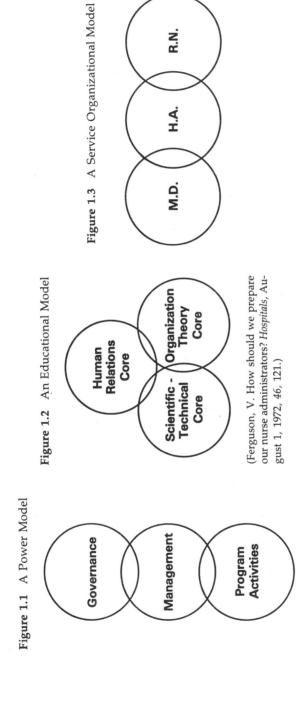

Figure 1.1 A Power Model

Governance

Management

Program Activities

Figure 1.2 An Educational Model

Human Relations Core

Organization Theory Core

Scientific - Technical Core

(Ferguson, V. How should we prepare our nurse administrators? *Hospitals*, August 1, 1972, *46*, 121.)

Figure 1.3 A Service Organizational Model

M.D.

H.A.

R.N.

11

instant substitutability for inadequate or absent support services which are the responsibility of the hospital administrator (H.A.) thwart nurses from perfecting their unique contribution to nursing care.

The skills of negotiation which embody persuasion and accommodation must be learned and practiced. Nurses must become and remain political as health care to people is organized, delivered, financed, and evaluated.

POLICY

The policy process is a conceptualized sequence of activities that can be categorized as follows:

1. Problem identification
2. Policy formulation
3. Policy adoption
4. Policy implementation
5. Policy evaluation

Some of the questions to be considered include:

- What is a policy problem? What makes it so?
- What are some viable alternatives to the problem?
- Who participates in policy formulation?
- What is done, if anything, to effect a policy decision?
- How is the effectiveness of a policy measured?
- Who are the influentials that will be contacted when a change or repeal of a policy is sought?
- What is negotiable?
- Who evaluates policy?

Many more questions could be raised as the policy process is explored and understood. The principle for nursing becomes: Learn where policy is formulated; be there!

THREE VIEWS OF THE FUTURE

The Institute for the Future, a Menlo Park, California-based think tank is a research organization specializing in long-range planning. In their ten-year forecast prepared for the Fifth Annual Corporate Associates Meeting in New York City in January 1980, the Institute forecasted four major themes for the decade of the 1980s. The themes were high-cost energy, an adult society, an uneasy society, and new values as shared preferences. Consider all four themes, with special regard to the new values and shared preferences characterized as diversity over uniformity, me over we, quality over quantity, and participation over representation ("Decade Ahead," 1981).

Rick Carlson (1982), a futurist, recently addressed an invitational conference of the National Commission on Nursing. He predicted a conserving society where stress on individual growth and human potential would be maximized, environmental quality and home and family life will be preserved. There will be positive regard for health. The present horizontal health care system will become a vertical one where a patient-empowering system would replace a patient-centered or physician-centered system. He predicted that in the hospital of the future, where most nurses will be employed, the hospital's primary business will be the provision of nursing care. Human barriers will be reduced as collaboration becomes more evident. Decentralization to units of smaller scale will occur. His cautionary note is ensconced in his forecast of a disciplined society since more discipline will be required to hold things together. A new conservatism becomes a part of the disciplined society, and with it, the recent gains made by nurses, women, and other minorities will be compromised as the new accommodation is sought when finite resources are acknowledged.

Health care of the future, according to Carlson, will advocate holistic care. As nurses plan strategically to enter and remain a dominant force in the power—politics—policy triad, nursing must take responsibility for its belief and practice of holistic care. Carlson's view of nursing texts written in this century as well as nurse attendance at workshops focused on holism, cause him to conclude that nursing is ahead of the future of the health care system; nursing probably does not know this nor take credit for it, according to Carlson.

At the Hastings General Meeting on "Designing our Descendants," MacIntyre (1979) listed seven traits to cultivate for the future. They are:

1. Ability to live with uncertainty
2. Roots in particularity
3. Nonmanipulative relations
4. Finding a vocation in one's work
5. Accepting one's death
6. Hope
7. Willingness to take up arms

These views of the future should lend direction to nurses as influence is sought. That influence is not for self-serving purposes, but rather to empower nurses to provide the best nursing care to the people nursing serves.

SUMMARY

John Adams, the former president of the United States, said, "I must study politics and war, that my sons may have liberty to study mathematics and philosophy. My sons ought to study mathematics and philosophy, geography, natural history and naval architecture to give their children a right to study painting, poetry, music, architecture, statuary, tapestry and poetry" (League of Women Voters of the United States, 1972, p. 3).

Presently, the collective achievement of nurses does not suggest our readiness to study the fine arts exclusively. Nurses of the 1980s and 1990s must study power, politics, and policy. This study must be supported with an ethical and caring dimension which is characteristic of nurses. A united and informed presence becomes a powerful force to assure nursing's deserved influence as power, politics, and policy conjoin on behalf of the consumers of nursing care.

REFERENCES

Anderson, J. E. *Public policy-making.* New York: Praeger Publishers, 1975.
Anderson, T. P. An alternative frame of reference for rehabilitation: The helping process versus the medical model. *Archives of Physical Medicine and Rehabilitation,* 1975, *56,* 101–104.
Carlson, R. The Invitational Conference of the National Commission on Nursing, San Antonio, Texas, March 22, 1982.
Cooley, C. H. *Human nature and the social order.* New York: Charles Scribner's Sons, 1902.
Decade ahead. A report from The Institute for the Future. *Washington Post,* February 15, 1981, Magazine Section.
Department of Health and Human Services. *The registered nurse population. An overview from national sample survey of registered nurses.* November 1980, DHHS, PHS, HRA, Bureau of Health Professions, Division of Health Professions Analysis, Report No. 82–5.
Ferguson, V. D. How should we prepare our nurse administrators? *Hospitals,* 1972, *46,* 120–121.
League of Women Voters of the United States. The politics of change. Education Fund Publication, 1972.
MacIntyre, A. Seven traits for the future. *Hastings Center Report,* February 1979, 5–7.

Moses, E., & Roth, A. Nursepower. *American Journal of Nursing*, 1979, 79(10), 1745–1756.

Selected Newspaper Headlines and Captions. *The New York Times* and *The Washington Post*, 1981, 1982.

Smith, R. E. (Ed.). *Woman at work: The subtle revolution.* Washington, D.C.: The Urban Institute, 1979.

SUGGESTED READINGS

Aiken, L. (Ed.). *Health policy and nursing practice.* New York: American Academy of Nursing, McGraw-Hill, 1981.

Aiken, L. (Ed.), & Gortner, S. (Associate Ed.). Nursing in the 1980s: Crises, opportunities, challenges. Philadelphia: J. B. Lippincott Co., 1982.

Consumer Views. "Respect is first demand." *Hospitals*, 1974, 48, 57–61.

Dowling, C. *The Cinderella complex.* New York: Summit Books, 1981.

Ginzberg, E. The professionalization of the U.S. Labor Force. *Scientific American*, 1979, 240(3), 48–53.

Hennig, M., & Jardin, A. *The managerial woman.* New York: Pocket Books, 1976.

Knoles, G. H. (Ed.). *The responsibilities of power, 1900–1929.* New York: The Free Press, 1967.

League of Women Voters of the United States. The politics of change. Education Fund Publication, 1972.

Maccobby, M. *The leader.* New York: Simon and Schuster, 1981.

Phillips, T. P. (Ed.). *From accommodation to self-determination: Nursing's role in the development of health care policy.* American Academy of Nursing, American Nurses' Association, Kansas City, 1982.

Nursing, Politics, and Policy Formulation

Barbara J. Stevens

INTRODUCTION

Politics and policy formulation are key notions in nursing today. They are so because of nurses' growing assertiveness concerning the place that nursing should hold in the health care system and in the larger society. This includes nursing's obligation to participate in societal governance, not only in relation to health issues but in all aspects of political decision making.

Nurses (as individuals and in organizations) have been slow to grasp the tactics, strategies, and facts of political life. But the last few years have provided encouraging evidence of growing political sophistication on the part of many nurses. New political behaviors can be seen in the workplace and in the political arena.

In the workplace some of these behaviors are:

- Directors of nursing have demanded and received titles, powers, and responsibilities appropriate to their organizational positions.
- Nursing staff have demanded and received constitutions and by-laws protecting their rights for autonomous nursing practice.
- In some institutions, nurse practitioners are reporting to and through nursing rather than through physician organizations or officers.
- Directors of nursing are forming corporate or consortial coalitions for cost-effectiveness in purchasing, for staff education activities, for meeting staffing needs, and for other activities of mutual interest.
- Networking among peers in the same institution and among peers in nearby institutions has increased, extending the available resources for each involved nurse.

In the political arena some of these behaviors are:

- Major nursing organizations now interface on the policy formulation level, either formally or informally.
- Nursing organizations perform watchdog operations, reacting when other groups tread upon nursing's domain or when they fail to include nursing in health care planning where appropriate.
- Nurses are participating in governmental bodies and committees that direct or affect health care.
- Nursing groups have been created for the express purpose of supporting selected candidates for public office where the candidates' stances are favorable to nursing and health care needs of the nation.
- Educational conferences for nurses are frequently devoted to issues related to power, politics, and professional image.

These examples seem mundane today, but most of these activities did not take place a short decade ago. This is not to say that all nurses now have a sense of the political. One still sees self-abnegating behaviors in groups of nurses, for example:

- Many nurses who wish to address groups in some public forum still shy away from use of microphones, assuring that the audiences, or parts of them, will miss the intended message given without benefit of available amplification.
- Nurses, when addressing a group, often do not introduce themselves, failing thereby to indicate what constituencies they represent or who they are.
- Nurses fail to use human resources at hand. They fail often to interact with speakers or noteworthy guests at informal times. Nurses flock together with old, familiar colleagues, leaving the invited experts to talk among themselves.

These behaviors, while still predominant, are not found in the growing critical mass of nurse leaders. This group of leaders has fast developed the requisite political tools in presentation of self and use of resources. These skills, once only exhibited by a leadership elite, are now becoming the norm for nurses in major institutional and organizational positions.

POLITICS

Until recently, most nursing politics dealt primarily with nursing's own internal, intraprofessional concerns. Failure to create channels for internal decision-making processes hindered the profession in its internal advancement and in its development of political influence in larger domains. These unproductive behaviors are now being changed by both formal and informal organizational networking in nursing. For the first time in ages, it appears likely that nursing may devise mechanisms for united decision-making efforts. When and if this occurs, the profession will have more energies to put into larger policy issues of the nation.

In any case, nurses have learned the hard way the need for coalitions to create power and influence. Internal coalitions as well as coalitions with other professions and groups are required for effective politics.

Nurses also have learned the futility of an "all or nothing" approach in politics. They have learned to compromise where it is not possible to achieve all desirable objectives at the first round. Additionally, they have learned to "count the votes" and recognize the futility of supporting bills that cannot be "sold" to legislators.

The State of New York, in its failure to pass the 1985 proposal making the Bachelor of Science in Nursing (BSN) the first professional level, was a case study for those who wish to learn from past errors in the political process. In the BSN controversy, nursing was its own worst enemy, losing the bill as well as much of its credibility with legislators. Not only was the bill opposed by those nurses who objected to this raising of the standard, but there was opposition by those nursing groups who thought the standard was too low. Additional opposition was offered by nurses who objected to the bill because it grandfathered present RNs into professional status.

These last two groups illustrate a political naivete that did (and to a lesser degree, still does) prevent nursing's political effectiveness. In the first case, the opponents (those who objected to the 1985 proposal because they saw the BSN as too low a level for professional practice) helped to defeat the first step toward that which they purported to support. In future negotiations, it is far more likely that nursing would be able to win advancement from baccalaureate to master's level than from diploma to master's level. In this case, the old proverb, "The best is the enemy of the good," certainly applies. Because they could envision something ideal, these nurses worked against a real, if limited, achievement.

In the second case, some nurses opposed the 1985 proposal because it grandfathered into professional status present RNs of any background. This opposition showed a similar lack of political know-how. No profession in the history of this country has been able to advance its status without protecting its present practitioners. To expect nursing to be able to do what no other profession has achieved lacks insight into both human behavior and politics. Even if one admitted the worthiness of the goal, it was illogical to think that the majority of the nurses in the nation would ever cast aside their own self-interest and disenfranchise themselves for the future good of upcoming generations of nurses.

And were all nurses somehow to support such a move, it still is unlikely that legislators could justify voting for a bill that reduced the status and productivity potential of approximately 80 percent of all nurses of the nation. Here again, an envisioned ideal (no nurse will be called "professional" without the required credentials) was supported in spite of the political reality: someone must have the authority to deliver care today in the existent health care institutions.

Such dissenters as those nurses cited above failed to differentiate between political decision making and intellectual ideals. Such political positions characterized nursing in the past, but the influence of such nursing groups is fast declining.

POLITICS AND TRUTHS

One of the major lessons, then, that nurses have learned is the difference between politics and eternal truths. Politics is the domain of practical decision making. It does not seek universal truths; it seeks the right decision for *this* issue in *this* political climate at *this* time. Knowledge of universal truths (if there be any) underlying politics may help explain past events or predict future trends. Such knowledge may even be useful, though not entirely directive, in making immediate political decisions. Knowledge of universals, however, does not assure right political decisions. One cannot compare an alternative foregone to one adopted. There will never be an arena where such comparisons can be made. Nor will persons ever agree on how the universal should have been applied in a course of action. Opposite conclusions often are drawn by various parties applying the same principle.

The best that one can do in evaluating a policy decision is to ask whether or not it achieved the objectives intended when the decision was made. Even where desired objectives were achieved, it is still possible that another course might have achieved them at a lesser cost, more rapidly, with greater side benefits.

In the past, nurses often have waited for some universal truth to shine forth or for consensus to be reached on a course of action. They have now learned that one cannot wait for certainty or even for highly limited risk. In many cases, nurses failed to act at a critical decision point, not recognizing that failure to act is itself a political action in the domain of practical affairs. This pattern of stasis has, until recently, dominated nursing's internal affairs. Now there are signs that that era is ending.

Most political questions do not concern themselves with truths, and nurses are misled in that they seek such truths where they cannot be found. Take, for example, the question of whether or not so-called technical nursing education is a part of or separate from professional education. Study after study has been done to see if one position or the other is true. These studies, ironically, seek to determine the impossible. The truth is that it would be possible to construct such programs (and their interfaces) in either model. There is no universal truth; there only are political decisions made as to what model is to be implemented in any given curriculum.

Politics deal with choices, not truths. Politics call for the best judgment possible in terms of forseeable results. Nor do principles—such as they exist—always help in the existent situation. One might, for example, postulate a principle that it is easier to upgrade a profession (with all the related costs) during a period of plentiful resources than during a period of scarce resources. Yet nursing failed to mass its forces to support baccalaureate education as the first professional level of practice when it had an economically favorable time. Now, it must mount that campaign in an era of scarce health care dollars, an era when it is difficult for legislators to support an idea that increases costs for preparing health practitioners. The principle (act when conditions are optimal) is self-evident, but it does not change the facts of the present national economy or of nursing's goals at this time.

POLICY FORMULATION

Given that nurses are improving in the strategies and tactics of politics, internally and on a societal level, what have been the specific policy successes? Nationally, nursing has not initiated any major societal health care policy, though it has reacted strongly (with support or opposition) to policies proposed by others. Support of national health insurance is a case in point. A more active and creative role in policy development should now be a goal of the profession.

On its own behalf, nursing has been more successful, keeping federal support levels for nursing high until very recently. Ironically, the growing dependency on federal monies created by this success may be detrimental in the present political scene. At present, initiatives are shifting from federal to state and local governments. Additionally, less external support dollars are available from both governmental and private sources. Now one must ask how rapidly nursing will respond to the changing politics. How rapidly can the profession make inroads on lower levels of government when its previous efforts were primarily directed at the national level? How will nurses manage in a competitive health care market when artificial supports for its services may be removed?

SUMMARY

Internally, nursing has been more successful in policy setting. The recent ratification of the National League for Nursing Board position on the baccalaureate as the first professional degree is a case in point. This action showed a united thrust by two previously independent groups— those in baccalaureate and higher nursing education, and those in associate degree nursing education. In addition to successful coalition support for a major position (an achievement in itself), one notes that this is the first time in a long while that the two major nursing organizations (American Nurses' Association and the National League for Nursing) have held in common a major position concerning the profession of nursing. Let us hope that this unity is a sign of future ability to agree on policies for the profession.

Let us also hope that once internal policies are determined, nursing will take on its full obligation in the policy-setting realm of societal governance. Things are improving; nurses are learning that one must function from the reality, not from the ideal. The cost of this lesson has been hard, but the profession appears to be learning fast and taking on the challenge of developing political effectiveness.

[2]

Governmental Perspectives

The Government, Politics, and
Nursing: Experiencing
Governmental Health Policy

Diane O'Neill McGivern

INTRODUCTION

The need for political acumen in the nursing profession and this author's lack of experience in political activities made the Robert Wood
Johnson Health Policy Fellowship a perfect opportunity to pursue a
leave of absence from academia. The Policy Fellowship was designed
to provide health professionals with political work experience as
legislative assistants in Washington, D.C. The author's assignment was
to act as a health staffer for Senator David Durenberger (R.–Minn.),
who was chairman of the Health Subcommittee of the Senate Finance
Committee. This Committee has responsibility for Medicare and
Medicaid entitlement programs. The largest federal outlay of money
for health is received by these programs. Senator Durenberger was also
chairman of the Intergovernmental Relations Subcommittee of the Governmental Affairs Committee. This Committee was examining the issue of federalizing Medicaid during the author's assignment period.

It is from this framework that government, politics, and nursing was viewed for this chapter.

Politics has been defined as the authoritative allocation of scarce resources. It is the process by which people attempt to influence the determination of who will get what in our society. Politics is the process by which conflicting demands and aspiration are reconciled and social needs are translated into public policy (Kalisch & Kalisch, 1982).

In general, politics is an inherent part of all activities and relationships, so that politics enters personal relationships, professional activities, and social endeavors. Discussing politics and nursing could, therefore, assume many different focuses; there is the politics between professional organizations, politics in state nurses associations, and/or the politics of medical and nursing staffs of large hospital centers. The focus of this essay is related to the author's area of interest—governmental politics. Governmental politics includes political involvement directed toward the formulation and implementation of policy by congressional and executive directives.

Many interest groups and individuals with special interests are realizing that a vote for a particular official is only one part of a much larger process of influencing decisions that shape the direction of policy. Organized nursing is one of the many such groups that recognizes the fact that it must become more politically sophisticated to compete for the resources and recognition that will help it achieve professional goals as well as broader social goals.

NURSING POLITICAL ACUMEN

Where is nursing in the development of the political acumen necessary to advance its goals? The author's evaluation of the situation is that nursing is relatively new at developing sound political strategies, despite the numbers of years nurses have been writing letters to congressmen about health and educational funding programs. The reasons for slow development have been discussed elsewhere in this book. It is perhaps more fruitful to discuss the things nursing needs to do to become more politically effective. The presentation will be outlined first by what nursing needs to do as an organized professional group and then, secondarily, by what individual nurses should be doing in the context of the overall professional movement.

First, nurses as family members, educators, and well-educated citizens should begin to promote a socialization process that ends the apolitical, noncompetitive traditions of women's upbringing. This behavioral background places nurses at a distinct disadvantage in the political arena.

Second, nursing's educational process must include two elements so far not developed in baccalaureate and master's curricula. Specifically: (1) an understanding of the health care industry, the factors which affect it, and therefore the forces which impinge on the largest segment of workers in the industry, which includes issues of financing, insurance, reimbursement, and cost benefit analysis; (2) facility in the language of the industry and business community. Nurses must understand the perspective of administrators, financial officers, and insurance executives, and discuss in a language that corporate and other legislative types understand what nurses contribute to health care and what nurses expect to receive in return. Effective use of these skills dispels the sense of powerlessness, promotes nursing goals in executive offices, and ultimately advances nursing's goals.

Third, as an outcome of number two, nursing must develop a visible cadre of leaders who are political and who look and act the part of the professional/business person. These leaders must come from service, education, and industry, and political activity must constitute part of their legitimate work—not as emergency add-on activity. Nursing needs to develop this group in order to generate commitment on the part of nurses and influential people.

Fourth, provide financial and moral support to individuals in key political positions, particularly when those individuals are nurses. In general, nurses in government are not responsible for promoting the nursing position. What they can do is respond to nurses and nursing with information and advice.

Fifth, broaden nursing's political base by aligning with organizations which share goals, have leverage, and have certain complementary resources. For example, there are several nonhealth organizations looking at proposals to contain health care costs, including the idea of nurse practitioners as appropriate providers.

Sixth, analyze a broad range of issues and utilize these analyses for the education of staff members, other organizations, and nurses. Prepare material which helps to characterize nurses and nursing as well-informed people. Help form a nursing political history of health issues.

As organized nursing takes the steps outlined above, the profession will be eligible to be a political group. With the background described in the profession's goals, individual nurses can move ahead in a range of exciting political activities. The efforts should range from voting to running for office. They might be:

1. Vote, not just routinely, but rather seek out candidates who are supportive of nursing and health care reform. Let candidates know that you voted for them and why.

2. Contribute time, effort, and money to selected candidates, thereby gaining entry to the candidates for future information exchange.

3. Establish relationships with selected governmental officials and their staff, providing them with issue analyses, position papers, and informed opinions. This establishes you as a helpful contact. Maintain contact on a regular basis with the people you've identified.

4. Organize contacts which can be made in the name of your agency or institution. This obviously enhances your impact since your agency represents broad connections, large budgets, and a significant block of people.

5. Establish a focus on political research. While there is descriptive literature on politics and nursing, there is little or no literature reporting research in political activity and nursing. Given this gap in research and the drive to expand nursing research efforts, it is tempting to call for the research to begin! This is a decision made, of course, on two levels— the individual researcher and the nursing research community.

What the individual researcher pursues is one thing; however, the research community does appreciate the need to utilize nurses' investigatory resources efficiently. There is already a great deal of research being done in fields related to this subject: research in political socialization, well-described in the Kalischs' (1982) book *Politics of Nursing*; research going on in women's studies; and historical research in nursing. These efforts already provide a wealth of research findings. Nursing should apply the work done by the researchers in these areas to effect a change in the political future of nursing.

REFERENCE

Kalisch, B. J., & Kalisch, P. A. *Politics of nursing*. Philadelphia: J. B. Lippincott, 1982.

Reaganomics:
Health Policy and Politics

Patricia Anne Jones

INTRODUCTION

There are two phrases that have been in newspapers, magazines, and
television news programs consistently during the past three years in
regard to the Reagan Administration's policies. They are: supply side
economics, and the New Federalism. The use of both of these phrases
represents a distinct political philosophy about government. They illustrate Reagan's approach to economics in the United States. Reaganomics has therefore impacted on public health issues.

SUPPLY SIDE ECONOMICS

Supply side economics embody an idealized view of the world where
economic growth can be stimulated by giving to the well-to-do in society. Advocates believe that if the wealthy sector of society is given more
choices through having more money and paying fewer taxes, and is
given more business discretion through government deregulation, then
extra money and initiative will be channeled into business and industry. Furthermore, it is believed that if the federal government would
get out of the area of providing social services such as health care, education, and social welfare, then the private sector would serve markets
now being dominated by the public sector. More money in the hands
of the well-to-do, less regulation of the private sector, and the government out of certain services would add up to renewed economic growth.
All socioeconomic groups should benefit because the competition in
the marketplace will make services formerly provided by the government better and cheaper than when tax dollars paid for them. It is also
believed that more investment and looser regulations will result in
growth that will provide jobs for those at the bottom of the economic

ladder. The key to this concept is that growth will provide new revenue for the government; hence, the concept of supply side economics. In other words, the benefits will trickle down and benefit everyone, including the government. Advocates claim that taxes can be severely reduced in supply side economics, and no one will suffer any harm from the reductions in government services.

NEW FEDERALISM

The concept of the New Federalism addresses the level of government (local, state, or federal) that should provide services not absorbed by the private sector. Supporters of the New Federalism believe the federal government's role should be limited primarily to national defense and foreign affairs. Most governmental domestic programs are considered the responsibility of state and local governments with the exception of Medicare and Social Security. These are considered insurance programs rather than welfare programs. However, even Medicare and Social Security have not been immune to the budget axe.

In short, the Reagan Administration believes that federal expenditures for social, health, and education programs have taken too large a share of the Gross National Product. While it supports the concept of a safety net to meet the needs of the truly needy, it has become quite clear that there are large holes in the net.

Children, for example, were the first immediate casualties of the gaping holes in the FY 1982 budget reductions safety net. Children were hit particularly hard by reductions in Medicaid and Aid for Families with Dependent Children (AFDC). In the United States there are increases in childhood malnutrition and illness with a strong linkage to reductions in Welfare for Indigent Children (WIC) and hot school lunch programs.

The bottom line is that the New Federalism embraces a line of thinking that there is no obligation on the part of the federal government to serve and protect those who are less capable of helping themselves. To the extent that such an obligation exists, the responsibility is passed on to the state and local governments, private and corporate philanthropy, and the religious community.

In a way, this philosophy brings us full circle. Government rarely gets involved in matters that they are not forced to get involved in. No one else is willing to address these problems. The government is not all that good at solving these problems. These problems are the most difficult ones that must be addressed by a society. The real question is, if the government does not at least attempt to tackle these problems, then no one else will.

BLOCK VERSUS CATEGORICAL GRANTS

The basic issues in the block versus categorical grants battle concerns the allocation of resources and authority between the local, state, and federal governments.

Categorical grants are individual, specific programs such as hypertension, family planning, health planning, or immunization. These are designed to address specific problems which are nation-wide in scope or provide specific services aimed or targeted at high-risk populations. The reason the federal government originally got involved in these specific health areas was that state and local governments were often unresponsive to the needs of the poor and minority citizens. Categorical grants are targeted to these needs. There were never, however, adequate resources available at the state and local levels of government to properly deal with these problems in the first place.

In the health area, the Reagan Administration proposed to consolidate 26 federal health categorical programs into two block grants to be administered by the states with few requirements. This consolidation was accompanied by budget cuts of 25 percent.

Congressional reaction to Reagan's health block grants produced a mixed bag of results. While Congress agreed to about $266 billion in health spending cuts over a three-year period under the Omnibus Budget Reconciliation Act, it gave the President only a few of the permanent changes he sought regarding public health programs. The Congress significantly modified the original Reagan Administration proposals. Instead of the Reagan plan of two block grants with no strings attached, the Congress approved four block grants with controls delineated and reauthorized many other existing categorical programs. Generally, the budget levels were cut by about 20 percent. This is 5 percent less than what the Administration wanted.

In addition to the block grants, the Omnibus Budget Reconciliation Act included massive cuts in Medicaid with reduction in Federal matching payments to states. In exchange, the states will be allowed more selectivity in offering Medicaid services to the "medically needy." Less publicized are the cost reductions in Medicare involving increases in patient copayments and deductibles. Other cuts include reduction of the 8.5 percent nursing differential to a 5 percent differential, lower reimbursement ranges for Medicare home health visits, and a reduction of the reasonable cost limits for hospitals. All together the reconciliation and appropriations provided for $3.5 billion reduction in Federal outlays for Medicare and Medicaid, plus additional savings in the block grant and categorical programs and, of course, health manpower education.

The concept of the New Federalism is something which has a direct impact on nursing and health-related programs. It is very important that we understand the issues involved so that nursing can take a proactive stance.

PROACTIVE POLITICS

The key to taking a proactive stance involves two important concepts: First, one must be able to recognize the issues and questions that will be debated and resolve them at the state and local levels. Second, one must ensure for maximum access and input of nursings' views in the policy development and implementation process. This involves everything from grass-roots lobbying to developing alternative proposals to be considered by key decision makers.

While a great deal of the public's attention in regard to the New Federalism has been attracted by budget cuts and consolidation of many categorical programs into block grants for the states to administer, the New Federalism concept goes far beyond that concept. The Reagan Administration has been taking many steps, across-the-board, to meet its goal of a vastly reduced federal presence in health care services.

While a lot of policy and structural changes have already been made in Reaganomics, they haven't been radical enough yet to alter the basic structure of the federal government. However, changes are getting closer and closer to such a change every day. Therefore, perhaps it is fair to say that while the basic structure of the federal government under the Reagan Administration has not been completely changed, it is also fair to say that the direction and course have changed dramatically, and still continue to change. This means that there is still the opportunity to impact on the process, and there is still a lot of work to be done.

In addition to changes that have been made with the implementation of block grants and other aspects of economic and tax policy, the Reagan Administration has thrown out thousands of pages of federal regulations, stopped enforcing others that are still on the books, and through appointments to important regulatory commissions—which the American Nurses' Association monitors very closely—it has begun to make significant political changes.

In health, the New Federalism also means:

- Benefit reductions and other changes in the Medicare and Medicaid programs.

- Promotion of competitive health care plans which have the potential of radically changing the health care financing and delivery system in the United States.
- Legal questions as to how entitlements or basic benefits can be cut without due process.

It also means:

- Getting rid of health planning.
- Eliminating professional standards review organizations.
- Phasing out health professions training programs in various areas of practice.

There are three questions that need to be asked again and again, with regard to the New Federalism.

1. What is the role of the federal or national government?
2. What are our national interests here at home?
3. What interests must be defined by the national government?

The author thinks that, in general, people agree there are many programs that must be handled exclusively at the federal level. These programs range from financing Social Security and Medicare to providing adequate resources for the health professions education, cancer research, and related health research.

Some examples which illustrate that health needs are difficult to delineate to a particular state or geographical area are:

- Provision of health services to migrant farmworkers
- Control of the spread of infectious diseases
- Improvement of maternal and child health care

While some form of block grants may be useful in some cases, there are many health programs that need to be dealt with at the national level. This is central to the entire debate concerning the New Federalism. Aside from which types of programs should be turned over to the states is the more important question of whether the states have the resources and the ability to take on these important responsibilities. Some states, largely those in the West and South, are very wealthy due to gas and oil revenues. However, many other states, especially those in the North and East, are being bled of their industries. Their tax base is declining too because of high unemployment. Unemployment in turn fuels the need for more social and health services. If those states which are in bad shape are going to be asked to finance health care, education, and welfare, then their remaining industries will be taxed at much higher rates. This accelerates job and industry flight to another, more favorable location. In many states, deficit spending or increased taxes may be prohibited.

The brand of federalism espoused by the Reagan Administration is being forced on the poor, women, children, the elderly, and the chronically mentally ill. In order to have trickle-down economics, there must be something to trickle down.

During the summer of 1981, in the heat of the budget battle over Gramm-Latta II, columnist William Raspberry wrote about the New Federalism. He indicated it reminded him of a new car which he had purchased some years ago at a time when Detroit was trying to be cost-effective. On the car was the usual new car sticker announcing all the features and costs of those features. Next to the radial tires was an asterisk with a note to the dealer indicating that in order to decrease shipping costs for weight, the radial tire had been removed prior to shipping, and the dealer would find the tires in the trunk of the car.

The Emperor may have no clothes, but pointing it out has been very difficult. The President's response to the charge that the poor and middle classes are being made to carry the burden of his economic reform is that this is untrue and the fabrication of Democrats. So, not only is the Emperor unclothed, he needs glasses.

NURSING AND GOVERNMENTAL POLICY

The health care system and the political system are in a period of change at this time. The opportunity for significant position change and redirection is wide open. Nursing can be highly instrumental in bringing about health care reforms. This kind of opportunity may never be present again in our lifetimes.

There are several strategies which nursing may wish to select. The most obvious, for a government relations structure at any rate, would be legislative and political strategies. Nursing groups need to get the message out regarding their concerns about the cutbacks in funding to the congressional and state legislative candidates. Nursing is becoming increasingly sophisticated in the political arena. Most of the state Nurses' Associations have started political action committees (PACs). At the national level, ANA established a department of political education within the center for governmental affairs. One of the programs of this new department is to identify congressional district coordinators in every congressional district. The coordinators are responsible for supplying the demographic data on their districts, identifying the nurse voters in the district, and getting that group active in congressional campaigns.

Working in a campaign is a mechanism which gives nursing considerable visibility. At the state level this can mean being recognized as a political force. Such recognition can ultimately lead to the appointment of nurses to various state health councils and commissions. This is critical to providing input into how health services and mental health services are to be delivered in that state.

The time has come to talk about nursing's approach to the financing of nursing services and the financing of those services as a cost-effective alternative to the current system of health service delivery. We must reexamine our historic posture that supports fee-for-service as the major thrust for reimbursement of nursing services. This is not to say that fee-for-service should be forgotten. However, given the current economic situation, it makes good sense for nursing to focus efforts on delivery models and the financing of the models. Fee-for-service is the one aspect of Medicare and Medicaid which has driven up costs phenomenally. What guarantees does the public or federal government have that individual nurses, reimbursed on a fee-for-service basis will not drive the costs of health care even higher? There are no guarantees, and perhaps there should not be, given the nature of a free enterprise system.

The challenge for nursing at this time is to design a cost-effective delivery system for nursing services that can fit within the existing systems of Medicare and Medicaid. The purpose is not to add on services, but to alter the delivery of services in a more appropriate manner.

ANA has developed a legislative initiative for Medicare and Medicaid. This initiative takes the concept of community-based nursing services, which are already covered under Medicare and Medicaid as well as most health insurance programs, and reimburses nursing services on a prospective capitated basis. Payment for services would be based on the diagnostic groups for predetermined populations. The nursing centers would be expected to provide services to two of three basic populations: (1) the regular Medicare Home Health population; (2) Medicaid well-baby services; and (3) Medicare or Medicaid populations with a high risk of institutionalization or reinstitutionalization. There is a high emphasis in this third population on patients with chronic mental illness as well as other chronic illnesses.

Although the traditional visiting nurse associations would be prime candidates for participating as community nursing centers, the concept is available to other nursing service arrangements such as nursing faculty practice groups.

The most exciting thing about the proposal is that it will provide for a reduction in Medicare/Medicaid costs by utilizing a capitated basis for payment instead of a per-visit and specific service basis. Secondly—and this is critical for nursing—it alters the delivery system by reimbursing for a diagnostic grouping, thus freeing the delivery of nursing service from the skilled nursing service listing which says Medicare will pay for dressing changes, catheter insertions, and so on, but not for health teaching promotion and maintenance which is the essence of community-based nursing services. Thus the opportunity for demonstrating cost-effectiveness becomes even greater because nursing can then deliver more appropriate services for specific patients.

In the future it may be that all organized nursing services can be structured in this manner, regardless of the setting. Fee-for-service is attainable through this type of structure on a contractual basis and becomes very reasonable as long as it is linked to an organized setting.

The New Federalism does offer the opportunity to open the health care system to competition. If nursing is to compete in the market, the profession must be very sure about what competition means and how we will compete and with whom we will compete.

Prospective Payment: A Strategic Plan for Nursing Power

Franklin A. Shaffer

INTRODUCTION

On April 20, 1983, legislation was passed that will revolutionize the American health care delivery system and its impact will be felt in every sector. On that date, President Reagan signed the *Public Law* 98-21 (PL98-21), the Social Security Amendments of 1983.

Public Law 98–21 is a milestone in the history of health care and is, in the author's opinion, the most dramatic health care legislation since the passage of Medicare in 1965. This new law focuses on prospective reimbursement policies for hospitals. The new payment system begins October 1, 1983. Soon afterwards every hospital in the country will be placed on the new system.

The prospective payment policy is based on diagnostic-related groups (DRGs). It passed through the legislative process with remarkable speed. The process took approximately one month. Three months prior to PL98–21, former Health and Human Services Secretary Richard Schweiker first presented for discussion the prospective payment proposal for hospitals. The speedy action in passing the new law can be contrasted with three years of unsuccessful lobbying during the Carter administration for a similar type of legislation. Achieving a bipartisan vote for passage of a new law is a considerable achievement.

There are several reasons that explain why Congress acted in record time. The first factor that contributed to fast congressional action was the concern over the looming federal deficit. Another primary reason for the fast paced decision was the danger of insolvency of the Medicare trust fund. There are many complex reasons for rising health care costs. Population changes, the effects of supply and demand, new technology, and intensity of service are major factors in spiraling costs.

REIMBURSEMENT PROCEDURES

Excessive increases in hospital costs have been attributed by many to the system of reimbursement. The past payment system was based on a network of public and private third-party payers. Direct payments by patients toward the national health bill were decreasing while private insurance payments were growing steadily. With the advent of Medicare and Medicaid in 1965, health care payments by public entitlement programs rose also quite precipitously. Health care costs paid by direct patient payments then declined further, resulting in an insulation from the "true costs" of health care services.

In addition to the above, third-party payers reimbursed providers on a retrospective cost basis; that is, providers were paid for reasonable costs after the service was delivered. Under this past payment system, an incentive was created for overutilization of health care services. The cost-based system, along with little out-of-pocket expense, combined to stifle patient demand and provider incentive for more prudent and efficient delivery of care.

NEW REIMBURSEMENT PROCEDURES

The prospective new payment system will markedly change the health care system from the way it existed in the 1970s and early 1980s. Medicare will set national payment standards in advance rather than retrospectively reimbursing a hospital's individual costs. Payments are then based upon patients' diagnoses or diagnosis-related groups (DRGs). The same diagnosis is expected to consume similar amounts of resources or cost the same to treat in all patients.

The Medicare cost data from previous years (prior to PL 98–21) is going to be used by the Health Care Financing Administration to establish a fixed payment rate per DRG. This is a new reimbursement system offering incentives for efficiency. Medicare will then pay a hospital a flat rate for each of the 467 DRGs. If it costs a hospital less for treating a patient in any DRG category than the Medicare DRG rate, the hospital retains the surplus fee. This is the first time the government has endorsed making a profit by nonprofit hospitals. However, if it costs a hospital more to treat patients in a specific DRG than the Medicare DRG rate for that diagnosis, the hospital absorbs the loss. There will be winners and losers in the new system. Some hospitals will be at financial risk for poor management.

PROSPECTIVE RATE SETTING

It is important to understand the components of prospective, as compared to retrospective, rate setting. Dowling (1976) notes that under a prospective rate setting system, "providers are paid at rates set in advance and are considered fixed for the pertinent period (typically a year)" (p. 8). The external authority empowered to supervise rate setting is the Health Care Financing Administration. Dowling summarized his concept for prospective payment in four steps:

1. An external authority is empowered (by statute, market power, or voluntary compliance by providers) to set provider charges and/or third-party payment rates.

2. Rates are set in advance of the prospective year during which they apply and are considered fixed for the year (except for major, uncontrollable occurrences).

3. Patients and/or third parties pay the prospective rates rather than the costs actually incurred by providers during the year (or charges adjusted to cover these costs).

4. Providers are responsible for losses or surpluses.

In summary, prospective rates are a means of exerting more external pressure in hospital activities and plans. It is a means of building cost containment constraints and/or incentives into hospital payment.

PROSPECTIVE PAYMENT POLICY FOR MEDICARE INPATIENT HOSPITAL SERVICES

This discussion focuses on the Social Security Act Amendment of 1983. Maraldo (NLN, 1983a) summarized the significant features of the Prospective Payment Policy, as discussed below.

Diagnosis Related Groups (DRGs)

The system categorizes discharged patients into 467 groups based upon the following criteria: diagnosis; age; treatment procedure; discharge status; sex.

Effective Date/Transition

Transition to the prospective payment system begins on the hospital's first accounting period on or after October 1, 1983. Implementation of the prospective new payment system will be phased in over a three-year period. In the first year, 25 percent of the payment will be based on regional DRG rates, and a 75 percent weighting will be based on the hospital's historic cost experience. In year two of implementation, 50 percent of the payment will be based on a blend of national and regional DRG rates (25 percent national, 75 percent regional); 50 percent of the payment will be based on each hospital's last experience. In year three of implementation, 75 percent of the payment will be based on a blend of national and regional DRG rates (50 percent national, 50 percent regional); 25 percent of the payment will be based on each hospital's cost experience. In year four, 100 percent of the payment would be based upon national DRG rates.

Payment Provisions

The national DRG-based prospective payment system applies only to Medicare and not all third-party payers. Amounts will be adjusted for rural and urban hospitals within nine census regions in the United States. Hospitals keep payment amounts in excess of costs and absorb any costs in excess of DRG rates. Hospitals will not be permitted to charge copayments and deductibles in excess of amounts now required by law. Rates are based on historical cost data and the annual industry-wide increase in hospital costs. Rates are going to be updated in FY84 and FY85 using the index of the costs of goods and services purchased by hospitals plus one percentage point. In subsequent years, rates of DRG increases will be based on the opinion of a commission of experts.

Capital Costs

Capital-related costs are excluded from the prospective rate. For the first three years of implementation, capital costs other than return on equity will be reimbursed on a reasonable-cost basis. For the first three years, return on equity will be reimbursed at the same rate as the average interest rate on the Medicare Hospital Insurance Trust Fund, which is down one and one-half times from the current rate, summer 1983. Beginning October 1, 1986, all capital costs, including return on equity, will be prospectively reimbursed.

Educational Costs

Direct teaching costs, including the costs of nursing education programs, would continue to be paid on a reasonable-cost basis and would be excluded from the prospective payment determinations. Indirect teaching expenses would be reimbursed at twice the amount of the teaching adjustment under TEFRA (Tax Equity Fiscal Responsibility Act).

Quality Review

Hospitals would be required to contract with professional review organizations to assess the quality of care provided, the appropriateness of Medicare admissions, and appropriateness of care to patients designated as outliers.

Alternative Cost Control Systems

The Secretary of Health and Human Services can permit alternative cost control systems if it does not result in greater Medicare expenditures above what the government would otherwise have paid. Other criteria would have to be met at the discretion of the Secretary. A waiver for an exception could be submitted to the Secretary.

Exceptions and Exclusions

Psychiatric, long-term care facilities, children's hospitals, and rehabilitation hospitals, and all hospitals in Puerto Rico and the Territories are going to be reimbursed under the previous cost-based system.

Physician Reimbursement

The Secretary would be required to collect data and to report to Congress by December 31, 1984, on the advisability and feasibility of including physician payments in DRG rates.

Davis (1983), from the Health Care Financing Administration, presented additional features in the new reimbursement policies. She addressed the following areas which are in addition to the previous summary.

Studies, Demonstrations, and Reports

Reports due by April 1, 1985 will include information on how cost data can be shared with beneficiaries in a manner that encourages savings to the prospective program, and recommendations on whether and how to include sole community provider hospitals in the system, and the extent of uncompensated care. An assessment of the impact of the system, recommendations for rate modifications, coverage of hospitals heretofore exempt, and inclusion of inpatient physician services in the system reports are due by the end of 1985. A report on state systems' experience with prospective payment is required in December 1986.

Safeguards to Quality of Care

To ensure that quality of care is safeguarded, a system of admission pattern monitoring to the prospective payment system is planned. Such monitoring is already part of the total cost limit program required by the 1982 law. For prospective payment, the medical review mechanism will identify unusual changes in the volume of admissions, case mix, total reimbursement, and discharge status, and will investigate the cause. In addition, a system of DRG verification will be implemented to assure that the DRGs assigned to individual cases are correct and not creeping into costlier classifications. Finally, the system will strengthen our hospital conditions of participation by proposing to elevate quality of care to a new condition.

OTA Prospective Payment Assessment Commission

The law also provides for a review of the prospective payment system itself by the Congressional Office of Technology Assessment (OTA). The OTA director is to appoint a 15-member commission of experts by 1984, including representatives of physicians, nurses, health professionals, hospitals, business groups, and others. The commission will advise the Congress and the Secretary on prospective payment matters.

IMPACT AND IMPLICATIONS OF THE PROSPECTIVE PAYMENT POLICY

Bisbee (1980) stated that changing to DRG-based reimbursement would involve a major repositioning of the "carrots and sticks" that influence hospital management policies. Thus, the prospective payment policy is expected to have short- and long-range impacts upon the health care delivery system. Some of the long-range impacts are going to be an extension of the short-range impacts. One thing for certain is that the health care system will have to change. The major impact will be that the new system will plunge health care services into the competitive business world. The incentives for efficiency, and the decreasing demand for inpatient hospital services, are factors that will be forces toward a competitive health care marketplace. Health care is the largest business in the United States from the perspective of expenditure and percentage of the gross national product. However, it is usually neither perceived nor spoken of as a business by the average American nor by many health care managers.

HOSPITALS AT RISK

Maraldo (NLN, 1983b) notes that because of the new type of regulation and anticipation of serious capital shortages, not all hospitals will survive the decade of the 1980s. Some will deteriorate and become obsolete; others many go bankrupt. A study conducted by the Health Care Financing Administration reported that about 25 percent of the nation's hospitals are in the red, and an additional 25 percent have minimal profit margins of between 2.2 percent and 2.6 percent (Davis, 1983). Facing a sizable capital shortfall with the advent of the new prospective payment system, hospitals will necessarily place greater emphasis on profitability. This new emphasis will require increased operating efficiencies and the ability to maximize returns. The hospitals that do survive will be those that are organized and managed as efficient business enterprises.

Johnson (1983) indicated that the general freestanding community hospital will no longer be the cornerstone of the health care field. It will be replaced by either a vertically or horizontally integrated health care delivery system. The vertical system will result from the evolution of community hospitals. The horizontal systems will result from regional and/or national hospital chains that are investor-owned or religious-owned. Horizontal hospital organizations are already growing rapidly.

It is estimated that 30 percent of all hospitals in the United States are part of a hospital chain (Johnson, 1983). Recent projections indicate that if the current growth rate of these chains continues, approximately 64.5 percent of all acute-care beds will be part of a chain in 1990. This is a 125 percent gain over the 1980 level. Johnson also notes that, by the turn of the century, large chains will become sophisticated, supercorporations requiring managerial skills that weren't envisioned in the health care field in the 1960s and 1970s.

The supply and demand curve has already begun to change. There has been a decreased demand for hospital inpatient services, and those that are available may not be affordable. The changing supply and demand curve will demonstrate competition and conflict, which will increase as the resources decrease. There will be winners and losers under the new system. The survivors will be those who adapt to the new climate and manage their operations efficiently. It has been projected that approximately 3,000 hospitals will close by the 1990s (Johnson, 1983). Local control of community hospitals will probably be transferred to regional or national corporate offices.

These changes will certainly have an impact on the players in the health care system. As has been noted, the organizations will change drastically; it can also be assumed that the players' behaviors will likewise change drastically; it will be an "era of responsibility and accountability."

IMPACT ON HEALTH CARE PROFESSIONALS

Boards of Trustees

The prospective payment has been applauded by proregulation forces as an effective cost containment mechanism and a fair way to balance the books. Diagnosis-related groups can also be a powerful management tool that will help hospitals work with physicians and employees to analyze hospital services and the staff's performance.

Boards of Trustees in hospitals, by positional power, will play an important role in the transitional process from retrospective to prospective payment. The Board will become more actively involved in running the organization and will hold the chief executive officer more accountable than previously. Resources will be limited, and survival depends upon managerial expertise.

The composition of the Board will change from the philanthropic or community-minded persons to more business-oriented people. There will be active recruitment to have successful businesspeople on the Board. Caution must be exercised so as not to overspecialize by appointing too many businesspeople.

The Board of Directors will need to be familiar with the new payment system and will need to reevaluate short- and long-range planning, as well as its relationship with the CEO (chief executive officer), medical, and nursing staffs. The board will need to devote more attention to monitoring the outcomes of strategic planning and marketing hospital services. The board can anticipate some conflict with the medical staff as controls will be placed on medical practice. The granting of hospital privileges to physicians will be scrutinized more carefully and the individual physician's case mix efficiency record will be evaluated. Those physicians who consume a higher percentage of hospital resources will be less likely to be granted hospital privileges. Physicians will also directly compete with hospitals by offering more services in their offices and/or joining in medical practice groups and setting up their own laboratory and x-ray facilities. This indeed will drain some resources from the hospital.

IMPACT ON THE CHIEF EXECUTIVE OFFICER

The chief executive officer (CEO) will face a number of challenges. The chief executive officer will need expertise in management skills. Hospital administrators will have to become a new breed, developing better financial, economic, and political skills than they have had in the past. So far, hospitals have responded to cutbacks with administrative patchwork. Hospital administrators have frozen jobs, cut back on nursing services, and transferred high-cost services to ambulatory settings. Creativity, innovation, and risk-taking will be required in the health care system of the future. Hospitals will have to diversify. In some cases they will be forced to establish for-profit centers that may not even be related to health in order to subsidize operations that are not self-sufficient. Administrators who can adapt quickly in this new arena will survive; others will be replaced.

Maraldo (NLN, 1983a) writes that hospitals will have to be well-managed, not just from the administrative perspective but from the clinical perspective as well, educating physicians and reshaping costly physician behaviors. Maraldo points to a comment by Bedrosian, president of the Federation of American Hospitals, which summed up the situation by saying the government didn't want to take on the physicians so they took on hospitals, forcing CEOs to take on physicians, thereby making changes in utilization. Since physician decisions determine 70 percent of how every health care dollar is spent, acquiring physician cooperation in cost-containment efforts will be the key to success for hospital administrators (NLN, 1983a).

Lindner and Wagner (1983) indicate that some CEOs have been accused of operating their institutions inefficiently. Some hospital administrators will admit that, to date, they haven't had the data to permit them to operate efficiently. This situation will have to change under DRGs. The CEO will need, along with all other managers, an informational system that will provide data on case mix. DRG encourages such systems since it combines clinical and financial data on one record. The CEO will need to develop a strategic plan and clinical budgeting in some cases for the first time. According to Johnson (1983), "Successful CEOs will need developed political skills. One highly valued skill will be the ability to negotiate and compromise among diverse viewpoints and still maintain progress. Such consensus-building skills require knowledge of who to involve at what moment, and how much to expect of each party." CEOs will want a management team that can scrutinize operations as well as turf battles, and initiate corrective actions to keep costs down without reducing quality.

Johnson goes on to say that initially CEOs might overemphasize the price-cost equation and lose sight of the need to balance economics, quality of care, and comprehensiveness of services. There may be a tendency to eliminate programs that are not making a profit and to cut back on labor, especially the costly professional staff.

Economic competition will bring about change in the relationships of CEOs to the board and to the medical staffs. Changes in the way of operations may not be readily accepted by either the board or the medical staff. For instance, physicians are not going to accept refusals to purchase costly equipment. In the nonprofit sector, the CEOs can anticipate resistance from the board as they approach them with business strategies to compete. Frequently, trustees serve as a social service to the community, and may not welcome a business approach. Further, competition should bring about an attitude change among CEOs in not-for-profit hospitals toward investor-owned hospitals.

CEOs operating in not-for-profit and those in proprietary hospitals will have similar problems, but in varying degrees. The CEO in a proprietary hospital will not encounter the negative attitude on behalf of the board and the medical staff towards the concept of competition and profit.

IMPACT ON MDs

Maraldo (NLN, 1983b) notes, physicians themselves will not come out unscathed by the new DRG system. Medical practice will be restructured to some extent as hospital administrators are forced to intervene in the clinical management of patients. She supports her position by pointing out that economist Paul Feldstein predicts increasing competition among physicians for positions in hospitals, as well as with other health providers in the future. As a consequence, he also predicts the further erosion of real physician income.

The medical staff must be educated to the implications of the new payment system; after all, the system is designed to contain costs and it is the physician who prescribes for the consumption of most hospital resources. The physician will recognize that his practice is being monitored and will need ongoing feedback as to what inpatient cases cost. The American Medical Association is cognizant of the fact that the new payment system will place controls on medical practice, and will probably encourage physicians to look to the system to identify areas in which they can gain positions of control. There is an increasing trend for physicians to become hospital chief executive officers. This is a position that can exercise power and influence.

Some physicians will aggressively resist the new payment system, while others will recognize it for what it is and work with it. Physicians must be actively involved in utilization review and the hospitals' quality assurance program. The payment system is not designed to encourage a lowering of quality.

IMPACT ON NURSING

Nursing, because of its percentage of the hospital budget and its labor-intensiveness, is usually the first area in which a hospital administrator will cut costs. Many key hospital officials have made public statements regarding the potential cost savings that would accrue from using cheaper labor in lieu of registered nurses. To cite an example, when the Medicare cutbacks began, National Medical Enterprises dispatched a team of corporate consultants to their 90 hospitals. The team discovered that a number of hospitals can improve their "effective level of operation by altering the mix of staffing" in the nursing department, largely through increased use of LPNs and aides instead of registered nurses. Superior Care, Inc. stated in an interview with *AMA News* that, to keep expenses down, Superior Care would use an increasing number of unskilled aides rather than LPNs and RNs (Shaffer, 1983). Eventually, they believe, insurance contracts will probably even stipulate the use of skilled aides instead of costly nurses. The nurse executive's relationship with the CEO will be strengthened once the nursing executive demonstrates that cutting nursing staff will reduce costs initially; however, it will not be cost effective in the long run because less skilled care or less care will increase the patient's length of stay. Length of stay will be increased because the patient's condition will not be observed closely nor will preventive care be practiced. It will also reduce quality. The future health care system will find that quality of care is likely to become its competitive edge.

Interaction between nursing and medicine under the new system can be positive or negative. On the positive side, nurses and physicians can begin to collaborate and gain an appreciation for one another's realms of practice. Nurses and physicians can cooperate to improve the hospital's efficiency by collaborating more in discharge planning and patient education. They will need to communicate better and in a more timely fashion on their respective treatment protocols. An integrated patient record system using a problem-oriented approach would be more cost-effective in patient care planning and treatment. The negative aspect of the nurse-physician relationship will occur with the oversupply of physicians. Areas of practice conflicts can be expected as physicians try to regain activities considered nursing that were previously within the province of medical practice.

One thing is for certain: the nurse is in a pivotal position to make the new system work. The nurse is the link between quality and cost. But first she or he must be able to identify nursing as a revenue-producing cost center, and identify areas of cross-subsidization and downward skill substitution. Shaffer (1983) has suggested a protocol for nurse executives entering the prospective payment system. His protocol includes the following:

- Identify the nursing case mix profile
- Identify the staff mix needed to care for the case mix identified
- Identify nonhuman resources needed to care for those patients

- Develop standards of nursing practice for case mix
- Identify nonnursing activities performed, Cross-Subsidization, and downward skill substitution by staff nurses themselves
- Determine which support services should be available on a 24-hour basis
- Utilize case mix to collaborate with admitting in assignment of rooms
- Assess work flow into nursing and what nursing care flows out of the nursing department
- Determine by case mix where decentralization can be employed
- Use the management reports to invoke cost consciousness on the part of nursing staff
- Use quality assurance audits to correlate length of stay with nursing cost
- Correlate nursing productivity and case mix; nursing needs to examine its productivity and correlate it with DRGs.

This protocol presents the major areas requiring in-depth analysis within the nursing department. It will provide some insight on areas that need an internal and external assessment.

Prospective payment policy may very well be the nursing vehicle for power if we accept the change, plan for the future, and identify nursing's value to the DRG world. Power in nursing is based upon expertise. Nursing can be system-smart in the allocation of scarce resources.

An issue that must be examined in depth is the identification of how profitable nursing services are to the organization. Profitability of clinical services will be an important issue under emerging reimbursement schemes.

By using readily available data plus a fairly straightforward analytical method, nurse executives should assess the profitability of their services. A major stumbling block for analysis of nursing profitability is that nursing has been and continues to be included in the typical hospital budget with hotel services. Stevens (1979) stresses that nursing must put a price tag on its service.

Shaffer (1983) notes that the prospective payment system can be the vehicle for doing this. The New Jersey DRG project attempted to put a price tag on nursing service by developing a cost allocation statistic for nursing, Relative Intensity Measures (RIMs).

Maraldo (NLN, 1983a) identified some major issues concerning costing out of nursing services. The principles should be identified and included in an accounting system that is negotiated with the executive team. Nursing's worth will be valued more when the patient's bill reflects costs for nursing care as separate and distinct from the hotel services. A separate billing for nursing services will increase nursing's internal and external base of power.

Therefore, the barriers must be overcome. Some models exist for costing out nursing, as Maraldo indicates. CEOs will be more supportive once nursing documents its strengths to the organization. Nursing must identify its cost associated with each DRG as well as the revenue generated within each DRG. In order to be able to function more effectively under the new payment system, nurse executives will need a knowledge base in:

- Economics of health care
- Fiscal management of hospitals
- Computers and information processing systems
- Organizational dynamics and business administration

The nurse executive prepared at the baccalaureate level will need to obtain graduate education in these areas. The nurse executive prepared at the graduate level will find local colleges and universities offer the courses either for college credit or on a continuing education basis. Continuing education programs in these areas are readily available at reasonable cost.

Nurses at all levels in the organization will need to develop these knowledge bases. However, those who need it the most now are the nurse executives and the first level managers. These two groups of individuals will be in the positions to effect the greatest impact. These two groups will be among those individuals held accountable for the survival of the organization.

The success of nursing under the new reimbursement system will depend on the managerial skills of the nurse executives. Like the chief executive officer, the nurse executive will need a power base built on expertise in political skills, negotiation, and consensus-reaching. Nursing management must know that the name of the game is cost-effectiveness; the players include all providers, payers, and consumers; and the winner will be the individual who knows how to play the financial game—achieving quality at an affordable cost. The nurse executive will realize that nursing can no longer afford to be all things to all people at all times. The nurse executive will indeed need to be a power broker. The strength of this power will be in developing a strategic plan, marketing, and budgeting on the major ingredients in a plan for power.

The nurse is the hospital's public relations spokesman on a 24-hour basis, providing the feedback loop in the communication process between hospital and client. The usual scenario has been that the nurse listens to the suggestions and complaints patients offer and in turn reports them to the management to deal with or solve. Usually there is very little follow-up by management. Under the new system, the nurse's position in the competitive marketplace will become a major part of the marketing of hospital services. The hospital's marketing plan will include provision for listening to consumers and nursing personnel.

PLAN FOR NURSING POWER

As part of the plan for nursing power under the DRG system, the nurse executive will incorporate all available sources of power, including coercive, reward, legitimate, expert, and referent behaviors. However, the power base for the nurse executive is grounded in expertise. Expertise will be what will move nursing and the organization forward. Expertise will demonstrate to the board of trustees, CEOs, MDs, and to nurses themselves that nursing is the link between quality and cost. Expertise will be the influencing factor and the competitive edge as the executive negotiates under the DRG system. It is important to integrate all of the available sources of power in the right amount at the right time.

Politics may be defined as the allocation of resources, and power as the ability to influence behavior of others. These two words are the basic principles underlying any strategy to survive and thrive under prospective reimbursement. It has been estimated that approximately 80 percent of the nurses working in the United States are employed by hospitals. In most hospitals, the nursing budget accounts for around 50 percent of the hospital's budget. Cognizant of these two facts, any plan for nursing power should begin in the hospital (American Academy of Nursing, 1983). Since this will be the era of management—because survival will depend upon efficient managerial practices—the nurse executive must be prepared to assume the management role. A plan for nursing power must begin with an assessment of the management activities. The tools needed by the nurse executive to develop a plan for nursing power in an economy of shrinking resources should include strategic planning, marketing, budgeting, negotiating, and futurism.

The educational and experiential preparation of the planner needs to be addressed first. The question must be asked, is the nurse executive prepared to assume this role in an era of responsibility and management? The educational preparation of the nurse executive has been an issue of debate for some time, and nursing does not appear to be reaching a consensus as to what should be the educational preparation of the nurse executive.

Fine (1983) points out that in most normative organizations, the usual method for bringing about change is through the education of those in authority in the organization. In the hospital setting, the nurse executive should be the person to institute change.

Poulin (1982) has suggested the major curriculum content for the educational preparation of the nurse executive. The American Society for Nursing Service Administrators (ASNSA) has developed a position on what it considers necessary educational preparation for the nursing executive. Most of the courses included in the ASNSA position appeared earlier in this chapter. The debate must end; the nurse executive must be prepared to function at a high level of expertise in the management world. If nursing does not solve this problem, the marketplace will; employers will hire nurse executives with MBAs (Poulin, 1982).

Hospital administrators are already voicing the belief that nursing executives need to be prepared with a master's in business administration. Many nurse executives concur with the hospital administrator, for two major reasons. First, many of our graduate programs in nursing administration are not preparing students with skills needed in the real world. Second, graduate programs in nursing administration require undergraduate degrees in nursing. The development of adequate skills is the area nursing educators need to address.

Poulin (1982) suggests that curriculum must be reshaped to include changes so as to provide for a firm theoretical base in administration and role theory, organizational behavior, utilization of human resources, and theoretical concepts in nursing care. Various components of the administrator role should be considered within appropriate learning and experiential models: for example, financial management, labor relations, political perspectives, and quality assurance.

Fine (1983) notes that across the United States, the crisis in nursing has been documented from every local newspaper to the official findings of the National Commission on Nursing (1983). They all point to the need for leadership in nursing. The Magnet Study of the American Academy of Nursing (1983) clearly demonstrates the need for well-prepared nurse executives.

Like the nurse executive in the service setting, the nurse executive in academia will share the economic burden. The nurse executive in academia will compete for resources with the schools of business. Poulin (1982) notes that ''the education of nurse executives should exist within the curriculum structure of graduate schools of nursing.'' She believes that nursing administration must be recognized as an academic discipline through the operationalization of nursing theory.

The nurse executive in academia must work with the faculty to utilize each credit hour to prepare the nurse executive for the DRG world. Currently, there exists a shortage of qualified faculty appointments for those graduate prepared nurse executives in the school of nursing's community. This arrangement is preferred over having someone teaching administration that has not had the experiential preparation. If a college does not have the faculty, it should not attempt to conduct a program in nursing administration. Just like its counterpart in nursing service, if it does not have the nursing staff to provide services, it should look at alternatives, even the option of closing beds.

In order to recruit and retain qualified faculty for nursing administration, one must compete with the service sector. Again, nurse executives in the service setting found out what competition meant during the height of the nursing shortage. Academia needs to develop a marketing strategy for recruiting and retaining qualified faculty. Timing is of the essence. If nursing does not correct the situation, the marketplace will dictate the solution; nurses will increasingly opt for an MBA.

The nurse executive will rely more upon his or her expertise in financial management and knowledge of human behavior and organizational science to negotiate the system. The nurse executive must adapt an organizational or a global perspective; no longer can the nurse executive focus on nursing. The nurse executive must be part of the management team with a management perspective focused on what is good for the organization. Nursing will advance as the overall organizati n moves forward. In preparing for the new system, it would be beneficial to examine what other nurse executives have done in states where similar systems exist.

Shaffer (1983) documented several changes that occurred in New Jersey Acute Hospitals following implementation of prospective payment. Some of the major changes included:

- Decentralization of authority
- Changing relationships among and between health care professionals with nursing surfacing to the executive level
- Medical staff more involved in the hospital's operations
- More accurate medical records
- Personnel becoming part of the administrative team
- Purchasing or sharing computerized systems
- Improving upon internal/external information processing

The nurse executive can draw from these examples as she or he prepares for strategic and marketing planning. Decentralization was one result of the New Jersey DRG System which will certainly impact on nursing; it will exponentially increase the nurse executive's power.

The nurse executive should be part of the executive level managing the hospital. This should not be too difficult to achieve since CEOs are already recognizing the need to have a skilled management team. The CEO also recognizes that nursing plays a key role in the transition from retrospective to prospective payment. The CEO also recognizes that nursing is the link between quality and cost.

The nurse executive will utilize skills in organizational dynamics, business administration, finances, and nursing theory to develop a strategic and marketing plan. Prior to developing the plan, the environment must be assessed. Levine (1978) discussed environmental assessments in his article entitled "Organizational Decline in Cutback Management." He suggested that the following questions be part of the environmental assessment:

- What is the mission of the organization?
- What are the priorities for the organization?
- Who are the clientele and what kind of influence do they have?
- What is the past stability of the organization? Has it and how has it withstood change in the past?
- What is the structure of the personnel system within the organization? Can personnel be reassigned? Are the personnel under a union contract? Do you have authority to restructure the personnel system?
- What are the causes of loss of resources and revenues (federal, state, or local funding cuts), and do you have control over or the ability to influence those losses?

The nurse executive must synthesize this environmental assessment with nursing, asking the same questions before any rational decision can be made as to what activities can and should be performed. This assessment forms the groundwork for the strategic plan and marketing process.

Strategic planning may be defined as the determination of future organizational missions, objectives, and necessary policies so that the basic purpose of the institution can be achieved. The nurse executive participates in strategic planning for nursing and the organization. Planning requires time and support from all levels of management and channels of open communication. Strategic planning coordinates the multiple long-range objective of the organization and establishes possible trade-offs between the strategic plan (long-range future of organization) and the operational plan (short-range objective of individual departments).

Strategic planning should be performed ordinarily in every organization and upgraded routinely. This is not presently the case in most hospitals. However, if nursing wants to survive under DRGs, a strategic plan is one foundation for survival. It will assist the nurse executive in identifying with other members of the executive team options available to the organization.

Planning will reduce future uncertainty for organizations, but will not eliminate it. Reducing uncertainty will help to decrease crisis management. The nurse executive, along with the nursing staff, must determine the range of possible contingencies and the probable response to each contingency. Kaiser (1981) suggests asking the following questions:

- What is the organization doing now (institutional audit)?
- What changes are presently occurring in the instution's political, economic, ecological, and technical environments, and what future changes are likely to affect the institution?
- What alternative roles might this institution play in the future?
- Which alternative future seems best for the institution?
- What should be done now to realize that chosen future?

Now ask these questions as you plan the DRG system. The answers will provide a framework for planning action.

Another major component in the plan for nursing power under prospective payment is marketing. Marketing is defined as the strategy for meeting customer wants and needs for products and services in exchange for customer resources.

The effective nurse executive must learn to market his or her product (nursing services) to a broad array of customers, including patients, physicians, chief executive officers, trustees, third-party payers, and legislators. A nursing marketing plan should consist of four steps:

1. Identification of customer wants/needs
2. Design of products to meet the wants and needs
3. Preparation of nurses to deliver the products
4. Creation of a demand for the products (nursing services)

The nurse executive must reach out and compete with others in the patient care marketplace. Others are very willing to offer nursing care services to the marketplace. Examples are patient education, home health care, nutrition, and weight control. The competition does not see nursing ownership on these services.

Kaiser (1981) suggests that the nurse executive preparing a marketing plan ask the following questions:

- Do you have a set of written organizational objectives?
- Have you recently surveyed customer wants and needs?
- Do you have a customer orientation?
- Have you identified your target groups?
- Can you describe your main product lines?
- How do you promote your products?
- Are you involved in the pricing of your products?
- Do you engage in product improvement?
- What is your distinctive competence?
- Who is your competition?
- What are your production goals for next year?
- What is your community image?
- What are your competitors likely to do?
- Do your superiors recognize your marketing potential?
- Do you have ready access to the institutional data you need to project marketing plans?

Once strategic and marketing plans are set, nursing should have good insight into where to go next. However, nurse executives must realize that in order to get there they should act as a power broker, intentionally influencing the beliefs, attitudes, and behaviors of others.

The hospital world under prospective payment will be a "negotiated world." Every player will be competing for limited resources. Negotiation is the process in which each party involved seeks advantage. Historically, nurses have been rather passive negotiators. The nurse executive must be a negotiator par excellence. Gone are the days that the nurse executive can collect staffing data and present the data to the CEO, who will then agree that there needs to be more nursing staff. The CEO, in turn, will tell the chief financial officer to increase the room rates.

The reality of DRGs is one flat rate per DRG. The use of money, however, is more controlled. If money is used efficiently, and a profit is made, nursing will be among the survivors. The situation will be one of tradeoffs and compromises. Nursing has not always been prepared to negotiate.

Kaiser (1981) summarizes principles that need to be considered in the negotiation process. These include:

- Know exactly what you want.
- Build your strength.
- Negotiate eyeball to eyeball.
- Don't oversell your case.
- Don't underestimate the opposition.

- Expect to win.
- Keep your guard up.
- Be reasonable in your demands.
- If possible, negotiate in your own territory.
- Always have a total plan. Don't begin negotiating until you are fully prepared.
- Always phrase your questions for a positive answer from the other party.
- Build a relationship.
- Don't be confused by decoys.
- Don't make promises you can't keep.
- Don't worry about winning and losing.
- Start out with the general and end up with the specific.
- Send a confirming memo.
- Don't negotiate unless you are in top form.
- If you become confused, quit.
- Don't be afraid of silence.
- Be the first to introduce major issues.
- Monitor the tension.
- Be courteous and respectful.
- Don't be sidetracked.
- If you "goof," laugh.
- Don't rush the other side.
- When you win, quit! When the opponent says yes, don't say another word.

SUMMARY

A nurse executive skilled in the negotiation process will prepare the organization to live and probably prosper under the new prospective payment plan. Nursing is the hospital's public relations to the community and the future-oriented CEO has recognized this fact. Nursing can be very cost-effective. The prospective payment system could be the vehicle for nursing to acquire its rightful position in the health care delivery system, if nurses are prepared to assume this role. The new payment system offers challenges and opportunities. Nursing and other health care professionals must accept the fact that the payment system is here to stay and prepare themselves with the expertise necessary to thrive in the changing economic situation. Expertise is power. Those professionals and organizations that will survive will be those that have developed a survival plan and have invested in a management team skilled to move into this new era. The successful organization will provide their managers with the authority and responsibility to do their job.

REFERENCES

American Academy of Nursing, Task Force on Nursing Practice in Hospitals. *Magnet hospitals—Attraction and retention of professional nurses.* Kansas City: American Nurses' Association, 1983.

Bisbee, G. E. DRG concept generates mixed reaction in hospital industry as research continues. *Federation of American Hospitals Review,* 1980, *13*(3), 6–10.

Davis, C. K. National legislation and regulatory action. Unpublished speech presented at the biennial convention of the *National League for Nursing,* Philadelphia, Pennsylvania, June 3, 1983.

Dowling, W. L. Prospective rate setting: Concept and practice. *Topics in Health Care Financing,* 1976, *3*(2), 7–37.

Fine, R. B. The supply and demand of nursing administrators. *Nursing and Health Care,* January 1983, *4*(1), 10–17.

Johnson, R. L. Era of responsibility: Competition challenges CEOs to be tough-minded and to take risks. *Hospitals,* June 16, 1983, *57*(12), 75, 79, 80, 82.

Kaiser, L. R. New success roles for nursing administrators. In *Challenges: Stepping stones to success.* New York: National League for Nursing, 1981.

Levine, C. H. Organizational decline and cutback management. *Public Administration Review,* July/August, 1978, *38*(4), 316–325.

Lindner, J., & Wagner, D. A. DRGs spur management-related groups. *Modern Healthcare,* May 1983, *13*(5), 100–101.

National Commission on Nursing. *Summary report on recommendations.* Chicago: The Hospital Research and Educational Trust, 1983.

National League for Nursing Public Policy Bulletin. Reimbursement for nurses in the primary care arena: A cost saving for health care. New York: National League for Nursing, November 1983, *1*(5). Prepared by Pamela Maraldo, Director of Public Affairs, NLN. (a)

National League for Nursing Public Policy Bulletin. *The world according to DRGs.* New York: National League for Nursing, March-April 1983, *2*(2). Prepared by Pamela Maraldo, Director of Public Affairs, NLN. (b)

Poulin, M. A. Education for management roles in professional nursing. *The Dean's List,* March 1982, *3*(4).

Shaffer, F. A. *An administrative protocol for utilization of management information reports: Case study, New Jersey DRG Project.* Unpublished Ed.D. dissertation, Teachers College, Columbia University, 1983.

Stevens, B. J. What is the executive's role in budgeting for her department? In *Maintaining Cost Effectiveness.* Chicago: Nursing Resources, Inc., 1979.

[3]

Power in Nursing

Power

Margaret L. McClure

INTRODUCTION

Power, as a concept, has been receiving increasing attention from the nursing community in recent years. This is a very interesting phenomenon and may, in fact, be an indication that nursing is maturing as a profession. Previously, many nurses were loathe to discuss the notion of power and tended to regard it as somehow perjorative and foreign to them as professional practitioners. In spite of this attitude, each of us in nursing confronts and deals with situations involving power on a daily basis and, therefore, we as nurses need to better understand it so that we may be more effective both for patients and for ourselves.

POWER AS A CONCEPT

In reviewing the literature, one is immediately struck by the number of important and fascinating issues surrounding the conceptualization of power. A brief description of some of these issues may prove helpful to those interested in the subject, particularly from a research point of view.

1. How should power be defined? There are many who believe that power is an overall concept that encompasses both authority and influence; others see the latter two as separate entities requiring equally separate treatment (Beck, 1982). Still others use the term "influence" when they seek to define power, as do Shiflelt and McFarland (1978) when they state, "Power is defined as one person's degree of influence over others, to the extent that obedience or conformity are assumed to follow" (p. 19). May (1972) perhaps gives the simplest and most straightforward definition in his assertion that "Power is the ability to cause or prevent change" (p. 99). Certainly such a definition lends itself well to empirical data collection and may, therefore, prove to be exceptionally useful to the researcher.

2. Does power include the potential to act, or only the act iself? For many theorists, potential power is a legitimate part of the power concept; for others, power does not exist in the absence of the powerful act. Debate surrounding this question is more heated than one might presume, particularly since it would seem that many individuals in our society are viewed as powerful even when they are not engaged in action.

3. Does power exist as an attribute of the particular person or is it interactional in nature? This question is closely related to question 2. In other words, is the President of the United States a powerful person unto himself or is his power a function of his relationship with other people?

4. Is power in any situation finite in quantity or is it expandable in nature? It is quite likely that this issue is one of the most important under consideration, primarily because of its potential impact on the exercise of power. For many years theorists dealt only with the zero sum concept, never entertaining the notion that power might be expandable (Wood, 1973). In 1968, however, Tannenbaum proposed the idea that the total amount of power in an organization need not be conceptualized as a fixed quantity and this led to the development of a school of thought that maintains that leaders who share power with their subordinates may, in fact, increase their own power in the process.

5. How should types of power be characterized and/or classified? Almost every author writing on this subject has utilized some form of scheme to describe the types of power, sometimes referred to as bases of power. As an example, one of the most widely used is that developed by French and Raven (1959), is a system involving five categories which they label as: (1) reward; (2) coercive; (3) expert; (4) referent; and (5) legitimate power. The reward and coercive groups allude to the ability to wield power through the use of rewards and punishments; expert power is derived from superior knowledge in regard to a particular matter of importance to others; referent power is gained through contact with or exposure to powerful others; and legitimate power is attained by the individual's formal position.

There are other related issues that have been explicated in the literature, but it would seem clear that anyone attempting to do research on this topic would need to resolve his or her own thinking in regard to at least these five crucial concerns before moving forward in the empirical realm.

NURSING RESEARCH AND POWER

One surprising outcome of the literature search with respect to nursing studies concerning power was the revelation that there have been so few in-depth studies conducted in this area. In fact, those presented in this book are among the few extant on the subject. Again, this may be a reflection of earlier attitudes concerning the topic and it is possible that such research will increase dramatically in the future.

Without question there are many problems that readily come to mind that would make important contributions to our understanding of this important phenomenon. Those nurses engaged in nursing administration would be interested in the examination of a wide range of variables. An example of the kinds of problem statements that readily come to mind are the following:

- To what extent does a formal leader's self-confidence influence his or her use of power?
- To what extent is turnover in a hospital nursing department related to the power of the various formal nursing leaders, e.g., head nurse, director of nursing, and so on, in that setting?
- What is the effect of differential power on committee decision making?
- What types of power are exerted by particular nursing leaders in various situations?

Undoubtedly a similar problem list could be generated by researchers interested in the areas of education or clinical practice. Each of these specialties carries with it its own unique set of power relationships and has therefore enormous potential for study and knowledge development.

In summary, the author's personal viewpoint is that nurses' increased interest in addressing the issue of power is a symptom of nurses' increased maturity, and even self-confidence, as a profession. In the words of May (1972), "the chief reason people refuse to confront the whole issue of power is that if they did, they would have to face their own powerlessness" (p. 21). Perhaps nursing is finally achieving a sense of its own power within the health care system today and is ready to deal with it on an intellectual rather than an emotional level.

REFERENCES

Beck, C. T. The conceptualization of power. *Advances in Nursing Science*, 1982, 4, 1–17.
French, J. R. P., Jr., & Raven, B. The bases of social power. In D. Cartwright (Ed.), *Studies in social power*. Ann Arbor: University of Michigan, 1959.
May, R. *Power and innocence*. New York: Dell Publishing Company, 1972.
Shiflelt, N., & McFarland, D. E. Power and the nursing administrator. *Journal of Nursing Administration*, 1978, 8, 19–23.
Tannenbaum, A. S. (Ed.). Control in organizations. New York: McGraw-Hill, 1968.
Wood, M. T. Power relationships and group decision making in organizations. *Psychological Bulletin*, 1973, 79, 280–293.

Women, Nurses, Power-Conflict: Competition and Cooperative Approaches

Elizabeth Dorsey Smith

INTRODUCTION

Since nursing is a sex-role stereotyped field, it is important to examine the concepts of power, conflict, competition, and cooperation as they apply to the profession. Power—the ability to influence or effect the outcome of an election or decision—is now being recognized as a possibility by women. Some believe the ability to openly exercise power is "unladylike." Others believe that women are progressively emerging as an important force in the public life of the nation.

Conflict may be defined as a force generated by individuals or groups who differ over an issue, resource, or the approach to arrive at a decision. Resolution of conflict is an essential transaction for individuals. Conflict can be resolved in a healthy or unhealthy manner. Deutsch (1973) has advanced the notion of destructive resolution and believes that competitiveness contributes to a destructive resolution. Competitiveness and cooperation can be viewed as two strategies in conflict resolution. Neither is totally inherently positive or negative, but each exists within the context of the situation.

Traditionally, power has been associated with men. The word connotes active behavior. Traditionally, passivity has been associated with women. These perceptions are altering slowly in the United States. Nursing is primarily a woman's field. Historically, nursing has been encouraged to behave in the most traditional female behaviors. It is essential to review approaches women are taking to reshape their image. Nursing should adapt these approaches to gain more power in the profession.

POWER AND CHANGE

Power and its uses are necessary to bring about change. Obtaining and/ or allocating resources are two activities which exemplify the possession of power. Women and men have frequently been observed to differ in their use of power and the dispersing of resources, both material and human.

Control comes from the ability to exercise the decision-making process with respect to resources. How women and men differ in their approach to the exercise of this control has to be examined within the context of culture. Are women socialized to cooperate and comply with group wishes more than men who are socialized to compete openly with one another for a goal? Nursing has internal value conflicts with respect to group and individual control behaviors. A question to be resolved is how the individual's personal space compares with the group's space. How, for instance, has the nonconformist in nursing been treated? Hedlund (1982) advanced the notion that women prefer a cooperative rather than competitive mode for resolving conflict. One wonders why this is so. If the cooperative modality is the preferred approach, why, in female-dominated fields, has so much internal conflict taken place? Perhaps this emanates from the discovery that women's work is less valued than that of men. In addition, limited resources are allocated to women as contrasted to men. Do women actually behave in the modality of cooperativeness that they espouse? This has not been adequately studied to draw reasonable conclusions.

Some believe that competitive or constructive conflict, as defined by Deutsch, deserves to be prevented to whatever degree is possible. This approach, particularly with respect to competition and competing, can be a productive rather than destructive experience. Finding the balance between cooperation and competition is difficult. However, where issues of conflict arise, individuals may seek a resolution via a cooperative equality response and may be unwilling to emulate the accountability so aptly stated by Harry S. Truman during his presidency: "The buck stops here."

Preventing destructive competition to "whatever degree possible" could be translated into "at all costs." Often this "preventing" has been nursing's traditional response to conflict without enough emphasis on its resolution. Conflict was to be avoided, particularly if the conflict openly contradicted the male-dominated position. Too many types of manipulation which have given the impression that nurses are mindless, lack decision-making skills, and need not be taken seriously have been used by men. For example, the use of the "nurse-doctor game" language which demonstrates that nurses can have physicians write appropriate "orders" without appearing to actively tell them what to do. Decision making, responsibility, and personal accountability are essential to problem solving on a small-group basis as well as within the framework of a large, complex organization. Most nursing is practiced within such an organization, and nurses need to learn strategies for problem solving within nursing as well as within the larger arena of the institution.

It is imperative for the author to comment on the state of the art with respect to women and their behavior regarding competition. Who really knows whether women prefer a cooperative or competitive mode of behavior? Under what circumstances will either of these two preferences be expressed by nurses? First, most of the work in psychology, particularly social psychology, has been done by males. It is well to remember that the nature of formulating research questions, suggesting hypotheses, planning experiments, and even theorizing about the results does not occur in a culture-free world. The scientist, even the most unbiased one, is a product of her or his culture. Therefore, it is important to remember that the description of the behavior of women is also culture-bound. Competition and quality of resource allocation is an interesting concept to research with respect to women. "Freudian theory

(has) also characterized women as less capable than men of integrity''
(Hunter College Women's Studies Collective, 1983, p. 15).

The traditional role of the woman in the home has often placed her in
the role of allocating the household resources. Take, for example, food.
Traditionally, the adult males of the household have received the larger
portion of the meat and other food, then the remaining to children, and
finally the woman herself. This scenario has often been a universal phenomenon despite the fact that women menstruate and become pregnant, requiring protein sources beyond those of adult males. This conflict between the woman's health needs and her social role within the
family structure has been clearly resolved in a mode of less than winner-
take-all, equity, and/or equality. The notion of altruism persists. To behave differently would imply selfishness and women are not socialized
to regard this as an acceptable behavior.

In contrast, however, is the classic model of female socialization with
respect to competing for male attention. In a world where women are
dependent on men, males may be regarded as the ultimate resource
to be allocated. The story of Scarlett O'Hara as portrayed in *Gone with
the Wind* most clearly demonstrates the notion of a powerful and driving competition for the attention of men, and in this case for Ashley
Wilkes. Little altruism existed, and the winner-take-all value was clearly
evident as Scarlett collected her men. This value persisted even when
she was unable to obtain her primary goal—Ashley.

The author believes intense competition exists within nursing, especially at the higher levels. Whether this competition is any more intense
or prevalent than in other fields—for example, business, law, science,
general academia, and medicine—is questionable. When the issue of
competitiveness surfaces in nursing, the notion of competitiveness
within the occupational group appears out of place. This behavior appears to dramatically contrast with the stereotypic altruistic image of
nursing. Some think nurses are passive, trusting, obedient, and—above
all—conforming. Competitiveness implies these characteristics are not
found in the active role.

Nursing has been on a pedestal for far too long; pedestals may up-
lift but they allow for little movement within the environment. In nursing there has been very little real power, and those who acquire it seem
to guard it. Recently, women have entered the public arena in droves
and are well-represented in the workforce. In fact, the majority of
women are members of the workforce. As this has occurred, women
have recognized that they must begin to network to promote themselves and their ''sisters.'' Nurses are just beginning to engage in this
in an active, deliberate fashion. Perhaps as nurses concentrate on this

strategy for promoting themselves, there will be less reason to question the importance of "in" groups and "out" groups and their competitive nature. Yet, it is necessary to most clearly understand that equality is not the norm in nursing. Efforts to promote an equality concept do a disservice to the nursing profession. Conformity has existed as a sacred tenet in the field for far too long. Nursing has the responsibility for differentiating abilities and capabilities among its members and projecting this to the public. "A nurse is a nurse is a nurse" is a concept that has been advanced too long.

POWER-SEEKING BEHAVIOR IN NURSING

Another issue that needs to be examined is the relationship of power-seeking behavior and nursing. Some may believe that there is an element of social unacceptability in the act of seeking power. Historically, the myth has persisted that women who openly seek power engage in unfeminine behavior. The women of the 1980s have been openly seeking to acquire power, particularly in the public arena through the Equal Rights Amendment and other measures of legislative clout. Certainly Florence Nightingale demonstrated the need for acquiring power in the public arena in order to provide skilled nurses in the Crimea, and she was chastised by men in her Victorian culture. There is for nurses—as for all women—an ambivalence about acquiring power in the public arena. Often, because of the ambivalence associated with power seeking and its acquisition, nurses choose inappropriate arenas for pursuing power. It is a fact that health providers have power over patients who are a captive audience in acute care hospital institutions. Why then are nurses so frequently engaged in conflicts with patients regarding this power when most often it does not enhance either the care delivered to the patient or the nurse's image? Occasionally, asserting one's power in this arena is a necessary therapeutic intervention. Does this conflict erupt because the nurse may really wish to engage other providers in a struggle but is reluctant to risk pursuing the conflict in situations not weighted as heavily in her or his favor? The conflict is played out with substitutes—the patients, not the physicians and/or administrators.

Nursing has translated the scarcity of its "real power" within the health care delivery system to the internal environment of nursing itself. Nurses badly need to applaud and reward one another for the variety of diverse contributions they make to the health care arena. Scarcity of contributions does not exist. Only recently has nursing made a move at many levels to honor its living heroes. This is a significant action, for recognition of one another is a deliberate strategy for empowering more nurses. Primary nursing, advanced nursing practice, political activity, and involvement of a multiplicity of nurses in the general health care delivery scene are important strategies for increasingly empowering individual nurses. More significantly, these activities encourage nurses to exercise power that truly exists. In the public arena, exerting power in conflicting situations may call for a variety of strategies such as competition, especially for the limited resource commonly called the health care dollar; collaboration, with other professionals to provide comprehensive services; and cooperation, in forming alliances for advancing our political positions. Most of all, nurses need to take credit for their activities. Invisibility has contributed to the public image of powerlessness. According to Kanter (1977), "the powerful are the ones who have access to tools for action" (p. 166). Credibility means power. "Power issues occupy center stage not because individuals are greedy for more, but because . . . people are incapacitated without it" (p. 205).

REFERENCES

Deutsch, M. *The resolution of conflict.* New Haven: Yale University Press, 1973.

Hedlund, N. Cooperative effects of competitive power conflict. Unpublished paper presented at the 18th Annual Stewart Conference, New York, New York, April 23, 1982.

Hunter College Women's Studies Collective (E. D. Smith, Member). *Women's realities: Women's choices.* Oxford Publishing Company, 1983.

Kanter, R. *Men and women of the corporation.* New York: Basic Books, 1977.

The Illusion of Power

Pamela Maraldo

THE PERCEPTION OF POWER IS POWER

When Jimmy Breslin (1975) described Tip O'Neil, Speaker of the House of Representatives, in his bestseller, *How the Good Guys Finally Won*, he stated that O'Neil had a great political weapon called power. O'Neil understood that power is primarily an illusion. If people think you have power, then you have power. If people think you have no power, then you have no power. So the idea is to get people to perceive you as powerful, which is not a simple task.

In the classical sense, power is conceived of as a Machiavellian control of the masses whereby the individual in power exerts a masterful grip over others who are less intelligent and skillful. Power, however, is not elusive. It pervades all human relationships, and is present even in the most common of interpersonal situations. Some are familiar with the enslaving power one lover can have over another. Romantic films and novels have depicted this human situation. Psychologists have asserted that deeply felt swooning attractions are based on a kind of power which is only perceived and usually has no basis in reality. The love object is perceived to have magical powers which may have little to do with the real loved individual. A smitten romantic falls desperately in love with an idealized version of the loved one, an image that represents a fantasy. The loved one, in turn, falls in love with the notion of being worshipped and idolized.

Another frequently observed depiction of the illusory quality of power can be seen in the dangerous arms race between the United States and the Soviet Union. To military officials the issue is not, as many believe, which country is better equipped to destroy the other, but which nation is able to project the greater image of power and strength and which projects one of weakness and vulnerability.

People with power know that power is mythical. It is created by impressions, perceptions, and illusions. Politicians call it the game of "smoke screens and blue mirrors" and they are masters at it. They live by the adage that it's not what you say, it's how you say it. Just as important, politicians know how to say nothing very convincingly, while conveying powerful messages by pretending not to hear or to be listening.

Power is the art of impression management. Power to influence others requires a high level of skill in the strategic manipulation of impressions toward others. Sometimes simply giving the impression of power saves the powerholder from actually having to use it. The threat to use your power to have someone fired or the promise to use your power to reward certain behaviors may achieve sought-after results without ever having to take action. Seekers of power who are skilled at cajoling, flattering, comforting, hedging, exhorting, exploiting, and exciting colleagues and higher-ups alike have an emporium of all the instruments they need to influence others. The powerholder needs to be equipped to evoke a wide array of human responses because humans are very complex and are influenced by different wants and needs. Korda (1979), author of the bestselling book entitled *Power*, points out that powerful people have the ability to dramatize themselves and their actions so that even the most unimportant events acquire meaning. Astute power players know just how to create and publicize epic crises in order to get the credit for solving them, and how to predict catastrophe just before announcing good news to make the good news sound even better.

BASES OF POWER: KNOW OTHERS AND KNOW THYSELF

Kotter (1977), describing the importance of power in organizations, states that the seasoned power wielder will often draw on more than one form of power to influence someone. This is necessary as a quest for power must usually be made on the basis of a personal appeal to the individual. A situation which illustrates this point is described below.

> One of the best managers in a company has lots of power based on one thing or another he has over others. He seldom, if ever, just tells or asks someone to do something. He usually tries to persuade them to his point of view. The power the manager has over other personnel usually induces them to listen carefully and disposes them to be influenced in a positive manner. He never risks getting the other person mad or upset by making what the other person thinks is an unfair request or demand. Coercion always invites retaliation.

Powerholders understand what makes people "tick." They seem to have a good intuitive understanding of the various types of power and methods of influence that will work in a given situation. They are sensitive to what types of power are easiest to develop with different types of people. They recognize, for example, that professionals tend to be more influenced by perceived expertise than by other forms of power. They also have a grasp of all the various methods of influence, what each can accomplish, and at what risk. They are skilled at recognizing the specific conditions in any situation and then at selecting an influence method that is compatible with those conditions.

The modus operandi used to acquire power in a university setting would not be suitable for the corporate world or Washington, D.C. because the personnae in each setting are different. Likewise, acquisition of power among staff nurses would require a very different approach from acquisition of power in a group of directors of nursing. In either case the motivations of the group, that is, what is important to each, must be kept uppermost in mind. To the staff nurses, career advancement and salary issues will carry greater importance than it would with the directors who are likely to be more concerned with budgetary matters or ways of dealing with the hospital administrator. The key element in developing a power base in both groups, however, will depend on understanding them and fostering an unconscious identification with those things that matter to them as power recipients. They must perceive the power seeker as someone that embodies the values they hold dear. In order to know what strategy to use to acquire power, the motivations of potential power recipients should be identified. Power is inseparable from the recipient's motivations, needs, and goals.

In this light, power can take the form of prestige, status, information, money, sex, affection, position, or anything else that human beings might be motivated to seek. There is indeed power in any situation. But in order to be successful in using power, one must have a sense of power. It is necessary to project an image of staunch self-confidence and a belief that others need and depend on you. Most modern scholars of power believe that personal strength is the most important element in any personal power base (Brouwer, 1976; McClelland & Burnham, 1976; Korda, 1975; Claus & Bailey, 1977). Personal strength is derived from a strong and realistic self-concept, which involves awareness of strengths, as well as weaknesses. A powerful person is able to withstand failure, humiliation, and a variety of crises. John F. Kennedy, during his presidency, referred to this characteristic as "grace under pressure." Herein lies the art of impression management and hence the illusory quality of power. Powerful persons have many of the same fears and inadequacies as others have, and they feel the same pain of failure or rejection everyone else might experience. They simply do not allow it to linger, and they never let it show. Power wielders exhibit an inordinate amount of control, and they always give the impression of self-assurance. They always appear to be in command of a situation—even when they are quivering inside.

POWER'S ILLUSORY NATURE
STEMS FROM HUMAN QUALITIES

Thus, despite its illusory quality, power is a very real commodity. Burns (1978) describes viewpoints on leadership style, as does Russell (Burns, 1978). Both men agreed that power is a fundamental concept in social science, just as energy is a fundamental concept in physics. Indeed, it is fundamental in every aspect of life. It is, in its most concrete form, the ability to influence or control; the ability to exercise sanctions. People in positions of power are in positions to execute their own will in a situation. Powerful persons control the reward systems and resources that others need, want, or desire. They are capable, as power wielders, of engaging in power exchanges that deliver things of value to power recipients. In turn, they receive support that may take a variety of forms. The power exchange may be political, where the power figure provides access to his or her staff in exchange for votes. The exchange may also be economic in nature where a hospital administrator gives a surgeon his or her own operating room because of the revenue that accrues to the hospital from the surgeon's practice.

But usually, at the root of any power exchange lies a very basic interpersonal situation. For example, a nursing dean might be very powerful in an academic institution because he or she provides a listening ear every time the vice president for academic affairs needs one. If the dean of nursing becomes the administrator's confidant, he or she has power over the administrator and over others in the institution by virtue of this close interpersonal association. If, for some reason, the dean no longer chooses to act in this role as confidant, power in the work arena may dwindle. The dean may choose to continue to give the impression that this association with the vice president is ongoing for some time after it has ceased to exist, thereby maintaining this power source. Others will likely continue to treat the dean with deference in the belief that he or she "has the ear" of the university vice president. It may be months before the dean of nursing is forced to relinquish this illusory power. Others will have to find out on their own that the relationship no longer exists.

The illusory nature of power is rooted in its very human, and consequently dynamic and transient, nature. Kalisch and Kalisch (1982) have asserted this quality of power in no uncertain terms. They think power is an inevitable part of all forms of human interaction, and that people (including nurses) who deny this basic fact will only find themselves at a serious disadvantage in making change. Power ebbs and flows in the interpersonal foray of any arena. It is subject to the viscissitudes of the human expectations and values that dominate it. Power is only acquired in relationships with others. It is always collective and never exists in a vacuum. For these reasons, power can be as temporary as a high school crush, or as enduring as a family tree.

Popular examples of the transient nature of power abide in the political fortunes of politicians and political types. Nursing lobbyists on Capitol Hill who wield associative power through friends and colleagues holding political appointments know the risk of having these power sources dry up when a new party takes over the government. If others know you have friends in high places, they automatically perceive that you are a receptor of privileged information and have access to very important persons (VIPs). Whether or not this is true is immaterial. You have power simply because people perceive that to be true. Politicians who hold high public office are vulnerable to the loss of power. It can be said that during his last days in the White House, Carter had almost as much power as the mayor of Dayton, Ohio. Many believe that at the root of Carter's loss of power were his failures at human relationships with colleagues, in the Congress, as well as in his own administrative branch.

A story widely told at the time of Carter's proposed hospital cost containment legislation should illustrate the point. The day before the proposal to contain hospital costs was to be voted on in the House of Representatives, Carter got on the phone himself to lobby certain members of Congress known to be undecided as to how they would vote. Making a valiant attempt, he got Representative Santini from Nevada on the phone, chatted for a minute as though Santini was his long-lost friend, then addressed him by the wrong surname. Slips of memory of this nature are unacceptable when dealing with the gargantuan egos on Capitol Hill. Santini is said to be the vote that lost Carter his hospital cost containment bill that year. After his power of authority and position were lost among his own colleagues, the American public followed suit in no longer perceiving that he exuded the confidence and strength that they expected of a leader. Regardless of his intellectual abilities, or his formal position as President of the United States, he was no longer perceived as being powerful. Kotter (1977) sums up the situation by stating that a person with whom a number of people identify is expected to act like a leader. If the leader clearly lets people down, the leader will not only lose power, but will also suffer the righteous anger of his or her ex-followers.

MANIPULATION IS NOT ALWAYS BAD

The most widely acknowledged types of power are the power of expertise, the power of association, the power of position, and personal power. All types of power are subject to the mercurial nature of human relationships. Powerholders—usually dominated by personal motives—draw from personal supporters, funds, ideology, institutions, old friendships, political credits, status, and their own skill of calculation, judgment, communication, and timing to mobilize those elements that relate to the motives of others they wish to control (Burns, 1978). None of these sources of power are infallible, however, and even though powerful people tend to develop all types of power there will be times when their sources are depleted or fail. Relationships may become strained or the expertise available in one situation is not forthcoming in the next. In any situation, power based on perceived expertise can influence the behavior of others as long as it continues to be perceived. Since information is a widely acknowledged source of power, the ability to act as though you have a certain expertise in a given situation (even when you do not) can also help one succeed in acquiring power. But there will inevitably come a time when an inability to deliver the facts will dissipate your power base rather quickly. This is risky business, but nonetheless widely practiced by seasoned power wielders.

Political scientists such as Robert Dahl (1957) have noted, however, that persons who are relatively powerful in relation to one kind of situation may well be weak in another. During these times the seasoned powerholder will project an image that all is well, that his tentacles of power are fully operational. This is accomplished with the utmost self-confidence that new power sources can always be readily tapped. A hypothetical illustration of this phenomenon can be aptly drawn from the political arena.

Lobbyist Jones from the American Nurses' Association needed legislative representative Dr. Smith from the American Association of Colleges of Nursing to "sign off" on a legislative initiative which Dr. Smith thought was horrendous. Jones decided there was no way she could logically persuade Dr. Smith because Dr. Smith just would not listen to her. With time, Jones felt, she could have broken through the barrier. But she did not have the time. Jones also realized that Dr. Smith would never sign off on an idea she did not believe in, just because of some ideal or favor. Jones also felt it was not worth the risk of trying to force Dr. Smith to sign off, so here is what she did:

- On Monday, Jones got Brown from the National League for Nursing—a person whom Dr. Smith respected—to send Dr. Smith two nursing research studies that were very favorable to the legislative initiative, with a note attached saying, "Have you seen this? I found them rather surprising. I am not sure if I entirely believe them, but still . . . ''

- On Tuesday, Jones got a nursing dean from one of the nation's most well-respected institutions to mention casually to Dr. Smith on the phone that she had heard a rumor about the legislative initiative being introduced and was "glad to see that the dean's group was on their toes as usual."
- On Wednesday, Jones had two faculty members attending a Washington reception stand about three feet away from Dr. Smith as they were waiting for the speaker to begin and talk about the favorable implications of the legislative initiative.
- On Thursday, Jones set up a meeting in Washington to talk about the legislative initiative with Dr. Smith and invited only people whom Dr. Smith liked or respected and who also felt favorably toward the legislative initiative.
- On Friday, Jones went to see Dr. Smith and asked her if she was willing to sign off on the legislative initiative. She was, and she did it. (Kotter, 1977)

This type of manipulation can often succeed when other power sources fail. It requires considerable time and energy expenditure, but a serious power seeker will use it, fully confident that there is always a means to accomplish an end and that he or she will always find it. But power of this nature is not a tangible asset. That is why power wielders such as Tip O'Neil assert that power is an illusion. You cannot learn to acquire power by rules; it has to come from inside. But some students of power, such as Brouwer (1976) and Korda (1975) claim that everyone can develop an awareness of power. This is the first step to acquiring power. Every person has power potential, but few use it or even know it exists.

THE NURSING DILEMMA

Nurses are said to have little power in the health care system. If you apply the power-is-illusion thesis, you could be led to conclude that if nurses indeed have no power, it is because they lack self-confidence and perceive themselves as having no power. Because power is ubiquitous and needs only to be used, a very cursory glance at nursing's natural power potential will lead to the conclusion that nurses are reluctant or fearful of exercising power, because all the makings of power lie

, within nursing's grasp. If you measure nursing's power by its expertise, or by people's needs for nursing expertise, a case can easily be made that great power potential exists. Everyone needs nursing care at one time or another in their lives. If you measure nursing's potential political power by the number of nurses in every state, there is also enormous power potential. Nurses are beginning to acquire power of position as well, evidenced by the growing numbers of nurses in high government policymaking positions.

This seems to be a paradox. Nurses complain bitterly of a lack of power in exercising decision-making ability, control of budgets, professional autonomy, and the lack of input into policymaking. So how can anyone claim that nurses have the instruments of power at their disposal? Or better still, how can one explain this apparent complacency on the part of the nursing community in the face of what one would expect to be a displeasing prospect?

Here is an appraisal: Nurses lack the most basic fundamental source of power, self-confidence. Projection of a powerful image of the sort that emanates from a sturdy self-image escapes nursing. Nursing lacks confidence in the value of the service it renders to society because it does not really believe that society wants and needs and is willing to pay for nursing care. An analysis of the power distribution in the health care industry leads to the conclusion that financial independence is essential for any provider group that wishes to acquire power in the system. In other words, if nurses are to acquire a power base in the health care system, they must obtain third-party reimbursement for their services. If one observes the first rule in acquisition of power, the motivations of power recipients must be identified. In this case, the power recipients are the consumers and providers of health care, who are motivated to receive and deliver health care respectively. In either case, these recipients depend on third-party payment. Consumers almost never pay cash when they make health care visits. The vast majority of patients have some form of coverage for health care expenses, and providers consequently need third-party payment to meet consumer demand for health services.

The road to power for nurses and the road to third-party payment for nurses are one and the same. And nurses have not, for the most part, achieved either, despite the fact that nurses have the potential power in other areas to acquire also a financial power base. Nursing has obtained some financial independence from the Rural Health Clinics Act of 1977, and some nurse practitioners are eligible for reimbursement in specialty areas of practice. Many in nursing's ranks, however, still do not sanction the practice of these nurse providers. Some accuse them of practicing as mini-doctors. Critics of nurse practitioners summarily dismiss them from the ranks of nursing, regarding them as physician substitutes, despite the fact that this preoccupation is counterproductive in today's legislative arena. In addition, this mentality which separates nurse practitioners from nursing's ranks divides nursing as a body politic, further weakening its power base in the legislative area.

In hospitals, the aggregate approach to reimbursing nursing costs frequently undermines the power of the nursing director and, consequently, the entire department. The profession has little power in hospitals because nursing lacks financial independence. Where are nursing costs identified in the hospital budget?

The key to acquiring power for nurses in and out of health care institutions lies in the hands of nursing's leaders and managers in decision-making roles. If more nurses in individual leadership and management positions had a sense of power as individuals, they could gradually succeed in state power arenas in influencing legislators to enact third-party reimbursement laws for nurses. Nurses would not, if power were an overriding motive, allow themselves to be diverted by academic discussions concerning nursing's identity. Rather than focusing on the differences between nurse practitioners and other nurses, or nurses and physicians, they would realize that as a body politic, their overriding concern should be to gain a foothold on power. To acquire third-party reimbursement is a foothold on power for nursing.

In hospitals, nursing service directors allow themselves to be diverted over issues related to the documentation of the true quality outcomes of nursing care. Many in nursing administration claim that in order to separate nursing costs in the budget under the new prospective payment system and consequently to gain budgetary control, studies are needed to demonstrate that nursing care makes a difference in patient outcome. In fact, if nurses themselves were aware of the fact that nursing care is a powerful resource to patients in hospitals (as well as the financial viability of hospitals) they would automatically move to establish their territorial imperatives in hospitals. Nurses naturally would then understand power and act with instinctive power plays and manipulative skill to gain control of their own budgets and that of the hospital administrator as well.

Nursing's long and drawn-out internal conflict over educational preparation for entry into practice is the ultimate testament to the lack of a sense of power it holds as a profession. A serious commitment to a quest for power would not overly concern itself with comparisons of competencies of the different levels of nursing. The facts are that in this society, credentials matter. Anyone who attempts to make the case that a college education is inconsequential for nurses is attempting to keep power away from them. At the 1983 convention of members of the National League for Nursing, a fairly well-known antitrust attorney who is not a nurse led a group of nurses to the gathering exhorting the nurses to vote down the League's position that professional nursing should be at the baccalaureate level. The gentleman himself has not only a law degree but is credentialed in the field of public health as well. It seems rather curious that an individual outside of nursing who tries to convince nurses that higher education is of little importance to the nursing profession, is so well-credentialed himself. If the attorney is as deeply concerned as he has submitted about restraint of trade in health care and the achievement of lower-cost quality care to the consumer, why does he not confine his efforts to the American Medical Association (AMA)? This attorney has written extensively on the detriment of physician hegemony in the health care system. He has not bestowed his efforts on the medical profession because, in an attempt to maintain their own power base, the AMA would surely not welcome the gentleman into their ranks. Medicine understands power.

Nursing must learn to use the art of impression management as well as the power plays that will succeed in convincing policy makers that nursing must have a say in how health care is delivered—in and out of institutions. But first nursing must perceive itself as powerful. A few nurses have learned how to project the illusion of power and to use the system, but most nurses are used in it. Kalisch and Kalisch (1982) have also pointed out that, as a group, nurses are underusers of power. Perhaps this is related to the fact that they have been a self-selected group with a low power motive. Only when nurses begin to understand that power is central to the workings of the health care system will they be perceived as a powerful force in health care.

REFERENCES

Breslin, J. *How the good guys finally won.* New York: Ballantine Books, 1975.

Brouwer, P. J. The power to see ourselves. *Harvard Business Review*, 1976, *54*, 66–73.

Burns, J. M. *Leadership.* New York: Harper and Row, 1978.

Claus, K. E., & Bailey, J. T. *Power and influence in health care.* St. Louis: C. V. Mosby Company, 1977.

Dahl, R. A. The concept of power. *Behavioral Science*, 1957, *2*, 201–215.

Kalisch, B., & Kalisch, P. *Politics in nursing.* Philadelphia: J. B. Lippincott Company, 1982.

Korda, M. *Power! How to get it and how to use it.* New York: Ballantine Books, 1975.

Kotter, J. Power, dependence, and effective management. *Harvard Business Review*, 1977, *55*, 125 136.

McClelland, D., & Burnham, D. Power is the great motivation. *Harvard Business Review*, 1976, *54*, 100–110.

Power in Nursing:
Group Theories Perspective

Margret S. Wolf

INTRODUCTION

This essay examines power relationships in nursing from a group theory perspective. The question addressed is: How can power be used by the profession to develop, grow, and maintain itself in its societal mission, rendering patient care services? Power is defined in this essay as the influence to bring about change.

SOURCES OF POWER

Wieland and Ullrich (1978, p. 248) describe five sources of power: legitimate, reward, coercive, expert, and referent. *Legitimate power* is the authority invested in a role or position that is accepted and recognized by the members of the organization. *Reward power* is based on the power-holder's use of rewards and benefits. *Coercive power*, the opposite of reward power, involves the use of punishment and the withholding of rewards. *Expert power* is founded on the powerholder's valid knowledge or information. The last source of power defined by Wieland and Ullrich is *referent power*, the attribution of qualities and characteristics based on some frame of reference, such as media image.

GROUP PROCESS AND NURSING

Before these concepts described above can be addressed in relation to the profession of nursing, it is important to take a historic overview of the development of nursing related to group process. One may inquire, can nursing be defined as a group? The author believes that nursing can be classified as a group using the following criteria developed by Loeser (1972):

1. Dynamic interaction among members
2. A common goal
3. A relationship between size and function
4. Volition and consent
5. A capacity for self-direction

Let us take each of the criterion separately. *Dynamic interaction* can be observed in terms of professional organizations and expanding numbers of professional nursing publications. The *common goal*, which may be subject to debate, can be viewed as the advancement of the practice of nursing—professionally, socially, economically, and politically. The third criterion is *the relationship between size and function*. This characteristic can be viewed as the potential power of over one million nurses in the United States. Another aspect of this characteristic is the current differentiation of nursing roles concomitant with the recent increase of numbers of nurses with higher degrees in nursing. *Volition and consent* can be viewed as the structure of the decision-making process within the profession of nursing. The final characteristic, *a capacity for self-direction*—a key concept for any professional organization— is a current issue being dealt with in the professional organizations which recognizes and struggles to preserve the independent functions in nursing, especially those associated with diagnosis, treatment, and health maintenance. Therefore, in its broadest sense, nursing can be viewed as a group.

NURSING POWER AND GROUP THEORIES

Two group theorists, Yalom (1975, p. 302) and Schutz (1966, p. 18) have independently described stages of group development. Through various methods of research, both Yalom and Schutz have identified three basically similar phases of human groups. These three stages are *dependence, control,* and *cohesiveness*.

The first stage of dependence is characterized by a search for structure and goals, a state of dependency and a concern with group boundaries. Despite visionary leaders in nursing such as Nightingale, Robb, Nutting, and Dock, nursing has had a long history of dependency in major decisions of health care. At this developmental stage of professional nursing, organizations were founded and university programs for the teachers of nursing were developed. Nursing education at that time emphasized the virtues of absolute obedience, selfless devotion, and a kindly disposition (Stoney, 1920, pp. 17–26). As recently as 18 years ago, Stein (1967) noted a fear of independent action in nurses in his study of nurse-doctor communication patterns.

The 1980s in nursing will focus on the developmental stage of *control*—a period of group growth which is characterized by a concern for power, self-determination, and control. In this group phase, according to the literature, differences in group members become apparent, with often contradictory aims and objects creating conflict. Intertwined with this phase in nursing's development are the influences of the women's movement which encourages assertive behavior and increased involvement with social and professional issues. It is during this current stage that nursing's struggle with the issue of power began.

LEGITIMATE POWER IN NURSING

Legitimate power—the authority of nursing to bring about change on the local, state, and federal levels—is an important issue for nurses to confront. The use of legitimate power is essential to the survival of the nursing profession. Trends across the country demonstrate areas of great concern for the future of nursing—for example, decrease in funding for nursing education; Nurse Training Act monies which require applications for nurse practitioner programs to be approved by the appropriate nursing and *medical* organizations; and nonrepresentation of nurses on health care decision-making commissions.

REFERENT POWER IN NURSING

Referent power already has been identified as a problem in nursing. So much has been written concerning the negative image of nurses that there is no need to cite examples of it. Referent power is strongly influenced by the media's portrayal of nurses. It is important to object to inaccurate images of nurses in the media and, at the same time, to emphasize in a positive manner the roles and responsibilities of nurses. It is interesting to note, however, that one-third (associate degree programs) to two-thirds (baccalaureate programs) of nursing students are from the upper one-quarter of their high school class (Knoff, 1972, pp. 371–375). One would never guess the intellectual capacities of nurses from their portrayal in books, movies, and television. Nurses are becoming more assertive: for example, they are more assertive on issues such as patients' rights, child care, and environmental health. Independent nurse practitioners are presenting a "new" image of the nurse as one who is accountable to the consumer of health care rather than to the physician or the institution. Nurse midwives and nurse psychotherapists are opening private practices and assuming full responsibility for the practice of nursing.

EXPERT POWER IN NURSING

The 1965 American Nurses' Association position paper—designed to place nursing education in institutions of higher education—was a decisive step toward professional expert power. The increasing number of nurses prepared at the baccalaureate, master's, and doctoral levels is a factor related to expert power and control. Nursing is beginning to view itself as a learned profession with the need to know why as well as the need to know how. The recognition of the existing levels of nursing practice with the identification of separate roles and separate knowledge bases is another step toward expert power. The recognition of the independent nature of nursing practice with its inherent rights and responsibilities—including accountability—is another essential move toward expert power and control. The consumer must be able to recognize and request nursing services based on competent practice and knowledge. Nursing, concomitantly, must be responsible for demonstrating its unique expertise in the health care system.

In terms of group developmental stages in nursing, the literature indicates that the stage of control needs to be traversed (not avoided) and the issue of power and control needs to be confronted. During the stage of control, there is a need to recognize differences. Much of the confusion in nursing today is due to the lack of differentiation in roles and responsibilities. Part of the confusion may be a result of the present licensure of registered nurses, a procedure which does not discriminate educational levels or prescribe differential roles and functions for the nurse.

STAGE OF COHESIVENESS

Applying findings from group literature (Luft, 1970, p. 28), one finds that when a group is able to confront the issues of power and control, it is able to move into stages of cohesiveness. It is during this stage that groups grow and meet their projected goals.

For professional growth to occur, the following four criteria are required:

1. *An Open System:* an increase in openness—that is, an increase in the range, diversity, and effectiveness of nursing's channel of intake of information from the external world; capacity to extend the scope of nursing's roles and responsibilities beyond current boundaries; capacity to change and accommodate new information and new clientele (for example, a focus on health maintenance in and out of institutions).

2. *Goal-attainment:* capacity to be flexible in goal achievement; capacity to seek alternative methods of goal achievement.

3. *Integration:* capacity to differentiate into subparts while maintaining collective identity.

4. *Pattern and Organization:* capacity to receive new members into the profession and transmit to them the profession's roles, responsibilities, and capabilities; capacity to formulate in a permanent form the groups' experience and learning and convey the profession's uniqueness to other groups (for example, professional independence in admission criteria, curricula, licensure, and decision-making power regarding nursing and health care).

SUMMARY

From the vantage point of group theory, nursing is leaving the stage of dependency—growing, searching, and forming professional goals. The challenge of the issues related to power and control need commitment and a professional identity. The success of nursing's efforts during this period of nursing's development is crucial to professional autonomy. The challenge belongs to us.

REFERENCES

Knoff, L. *From student to RN.* Bethesda, Md.: DHEW, 1972.

Loeser, L. *International Journal of Group Psychotherapy,* 1957, *VII*(1), 5–19. In W. M. Lifton (Ed.), *Group: Facilitating individual growth and societal change.* New York: John Wiley, 1972.

Luft, J. *Group processes: An introduction to group dynamics.* Palo Alto, California: Mayfield, 1970.

Schutz, W. C. *F.I.R.O.: A three-dimensional theory of interpersonal behavior: The interpersonal world.* Palo Alto, California: Science and Behavior Books, 1966.

Stein, L. The doctor-nurse game. *Archives of General Psychiatry,* 1967, *16,* 699–700.

Stoney, E. *Practical points in nursing.* Philadelphia: W. B. Saunders, 1920.

Wieland, G. F., & Ullrich, R. A. *Organizations: Behavior, design, and change.* Homewood, Illinois: Richard D. Irwin, 1976.

Yalom, I. D. *The theory and practice of group psychotherapy.* New York: Basic Books, 1975.

Power, Possibility, and Responsibility

Valentina Harrell

The images associated with a young child's mastery of the highly complex skill of riding a bicycle might serve as a metaphor to aid in our understanding of where nursing is today and where nursing is going. Imagine the intense concentration the child initially directs to mounting and negotiating the multiple, simultaneous maneuvers required to keep this contraption perpendicular to the ground and in forward motion—but not too fast or out of control, that is, in danger of total disintegration. At the point of the initial exhiliarating taste of success, the child exclaims, "Look at me! I'm doing it!" However, at the precise instant that Mom or Dad direct attention to the event, the awesome sense of power and a simultaneous rush of self-consciousness contribute to a catastrophic collapse of the entire venture. Until the experience of mastery is well enough integrated and automatic, calling attention to success can set up a feedback loop that results in sabotage.

The forward movement of the profession of nursing has gone beyond the requisite level of integration and solidarity, such that, to look at it and label it will not risk the collapse of the venture. Rather, acknowledging the power of the forward thrust within the profession is more likely to increase our collective capacity to identify the possibilities for the future and increase our ability to respond by directing the "vehicle" where nursing wants and needs to go.

As Ferguson (Chapter 1, this volume) has indicated, executive function is most clearly exemplified by the capacity to make decisions and plan for the achievement of long-range goals. Attention in the profession no longer need be directed entirely to the task of "keeping perpendicular." Attention correctly has shifted to what is ahead on the road as nursing moves towards increasing levels of independence, autonomy, and accountability as a profession.

In his latest book, *Freedom and Destiny*, May (1981) points out that "possibility" comes from the Latin *posse*, "to be able," which is also the original root of our word *power*. When responsibility is understood within the Gestalt therapy frame of reference developed by yet another existential therapist, Fritz Perls, the linkage among the three words in the title of this essay becomes apparent—"to be responsible," according to Perls, means "to be able to respond," or "to be capable of response" (1969).

May (1981), consistent with his humanist/existentialist world view, goes beyond pointing out the inseparability of freedom and responsibility. He adds, "Freedom is more than a value itself; it underlies the possibility of valuing; it is basic to our capacity to value" (p. 6). Attention paid to our "capacity to value" as individuals within the nursing profession and as a unified profession is well spent since this theme is intricately related to those of power, possibilities, and responsibility.

Ferguson referred to current shifts and transformations in our adult society of today resulting in the emergence of new sets of values. She suggests that nursing needs to "buy in" to the new value system. Nursing should, however, be aware of the fine line between "buying in" and "selling out." Perhaps in addition to capitalizing on the emerging values that are consistent with the dominant values of the nursing profession, nursing needs to accept increasing responsibility for the shaping of the values that are emerging.

Two shifts in values identified by Ferguson were from focus on quantity to quality and from representation to participation. Let us examine our response to two relatively recent developments that reflect these shifts in values: (1) the emergence of consumerism with the concomitant increase in public demand for participation and quality in health care; and (2) the emergence of health psychology as a branch of yet another discipline tromping into the territory of patient education and espousing the principles of participation and wholism. For some nurses there is temptation to withdraw, licking wounds and complaining, "But we have been saying these things all along. How come no one listened to us?" At the other end of the continuum are nurses who champion the cause of rights and responsibilities of whole persons and who fulfill their role as patient advocates.

Nurses want to be heard and want their contributions to be more evident and acknowledged, but who is responsible for whether or not nurses are recognized? Nursing should increase as a profession the capacity to deliver messages that get through to the right audiences. Volume, influenced by rage, frequently garbles the message, and withdrawal obviously negates any *possibility* of being heard and being in the position *to be able to respond*.

If nurses are not heard the first time, they need to say it again—and again—and again—while at the same time going beyond mere repetition to find innovative ways of packaging and merchandising the message to ensure that it is heard. On these levels, "buying in" simply means going along with what nursing has been doing anyway; however, with continued efforts to grow and expand the sphere of influence, nursing can really do it better.

On the other hand, in reference to another emerging value identified by Ferguson, that is, the shift from the focus of "we" to "me," nursing should consider a judicious combination of "buying in" with "holding out." Rugged individualism as a key to understanding the American character infuses all people with a certain esprit de corps. However, the need for balance between the seemingly contradictory values of individualism and interdependence must be acknowledged. Nursing's capacity for collective joining and collaboration for the benefit of the "we" is all too often devalued in the face of a felt need to "buy in" to the values of the "get-ahead generation." Whether the sellout occurs within the profession or among the peoples of the world, the potential consequences are frighteningly devastating. If the planet does not survive, what does getting ahead mean anyway?

Nursing's role as a predominantly woman's profession may be to use power and influence to contribute to bringing about change in some of the long-held beliefs and values that persist even in the currently emerging transformed society. According to Fiske (1981), women in research and academic life across disciplines have begun the process of infiltration and influence. Several years ago strategists in the women's movement changed their emphasis from setting up separate courses in women's studies to "mainstreaming" or pushing to incorporate material on the experience of and research about women into regular programs. Intradisciplinary ripples have already been felt (for example in psychology, political science, philosophy, the humanities, and others). More important, however, influence is being brought to bear on major relevant topics and issues across disciplines. Questions have been raised regarding the prevailing definitions of what is worthy of scholarly interest and analysis. Furthermore, increasing attention is being paid to the notion of what constitutes the appropriate methods of inquiry.

In a recent article in the *Association of Women in Psychology Newsletter* ("Dilemmas," 1982), questions were raised regarding what is being called the "feminist methodology." As described, this research methodology includes procedures such as collaboration, the study of whole people in context, and the tapping of their experience of the world. Is this really a new idea or is it more correctly a rediscovery of humanistic research, a thread which has already run through many disciplines and is certainly increasingly being talked about in nursing? The question is not so much the value of traditional modes of scientific inquiry over the nontraditional feminist-humanistic-qualitative modes. More to the point is the relative value of each.

The qualitative research presented by O'Connor (Chapter 7, this volume) has generated preliminary findings that matter—that is, that reflect a shared and relevant meaning. Such findings may have value that goes beyond p values of whatever magnitude, despite obvious and identifiable weaknesses in control and violations of traditional empirical research design. (No one would argue that a return rate of 10 percent on reports of critical incidents is problematic.) Nevertheless, the emergence of anger as a dominant theme in the secondary analysis of the critical incidents provokes haunting and lingering aftereffects. It seems like nursing "knew that already" and yet the finding resonates with a current that runs deep and consistent throughout the field and speaks poignantly to one of the major issues that influence the effectiveness of leadership and executive function in our profession.

How often has anger had a crippling effect on individual and collective *capacity to respond*? Indeed, the anger frequently does get expressed, but how often only behind closed doors, to friends, colleagues, family, or others who have nothing to do with the immediate situation? How often is it expressed in a self-sabotaging way via indirect action such as leaving the field or taking pot shots or mounting skirmishes from the bushes when professional decisions have been made that "didn't go the way a person wanted?" Attempts to influence without assuming the responsibility for staying in the field result in loss rather than gain in professional power.

Thus, the problem is not one of the ability to be angry or even one of the ability to express angry feelings but rather one of being able to respond effectively within the field rather than "being forced" to leave the field. (One is tempted to ask, "Forced? By whom?") When this "leaving the field" is generalized beyond the specific critical incident—possibly to that associated with burnout and the exodus from the profession—the potential relevance of O'Connor's finding becomes more apparent given the relationship of this phenomenon to our current major professional problems of shortage, turnover, and retention.

The profession is learning these lessons as the profession matures and grows and, in so doing, is gaining substantially in professional power. Thus, without risking a precipitous collapse of the venture, the author would encourage more than a cautious sideways glance at the ample evidence of nursing's gradually increasing professional autonomy, independence, and capacity for accountability. "Look at us. We are doing it! We just need to keep peddling because nursing has not yet gotten to where nursing needs to go."

REFERENCES

Dilemmas in feminist methodology. *Association of Women in Psychology News-letter*, March-April, 1982, 3; 8; 10.

Ferguson, V. Power, politics, and policy in nursing. In R. R. Wieczorek (Ed.), *Power, Politics, and Policy in Nursing*. New York: Springer Publishing Company, 1984.

Fiske, E. B. Scholars face a challenge by feminist: Women's research challenges long-held beliefs. *New York Times*, November 23, 1981, pp. 1; B6.

May, R. *Freedom and destiny*. New York: W. W. Norton & Company, 1981.

O'Connor, A. Continuing education, the power of nursing's leader elite. In R. R. Wieczorek (Ed.), *Power, Politics, and Policy in Nursing*. New York: Springer Publishing Company, 1984.

Perls, F. S. *Gestalt therapy verbatim*. Lafayette, California: Real People Press, 1969.

Career- Versus Job-Orientation: A Power Dilemma in Nursing and Feminism

Elizabeth Dorsey Smith

INTRODUCTION

In the 1980s, nursing is faced with a dilemma regarding the status of nurses in the marketplace. Nursing numbers are significant but numbers alone do not make a significant impact on the health care delivery system. The population of nursing is approximately 95 percent female. It is composed of women who have chosen the profession as a career and those who have chosen nursing as a job. McClure (1980) refers to this dichotomy as the white collar and blue collar nurses.

The job-oriented nurse is more likely to be singularly invested in the job which she fills and the income she derives from the job. This is not meant to imply that the career-oriented nurse is less interested in her remuneration; however, it is not the only factor considered in job satisfaction. The job nurse has been referred to as the "appliance nurse" who works to enhance the family income. Nevertheless, the job is seen as an end unto itself and efforts to become involved in professional nursing issues both on or off the job are minimal. Job-oriented nurses are more comfortable with very structured employment boundaries prescribed for their role and relate to others within the confines of these structured boundaries. Some refer to these nurses as ones who are considered more traditional with respect to the female role.

The career-oriented nurse is a person with the professional values of a continuing commitment to extending the responsibility for her own nursing actions and to acquiring new knowledge and skills which broaden her power base. The career nurse is frequently associated with feminism. This type of nurse works for the goals of the women's movement as expressed succinctly in the denied Equal Rights Amendment: "Equality of rights under the law shall not be denied or abridged by the United States or by any state on account of sex."

Career professional nurses are sensitive to the issue of equal pay for comparable work sought by Nurse Inc. in Denver, which sued for a pay scale based on this principle. This was the first woman's case to challenge the notion of pay discrimination on the basis of sex-segregated occupations, and the ruling—even though it was not won—paved the way for future suits which are only now having some success; for example, the Gunther decision which brought about pay equity between female jail matrons and male jailers. Before cheering at the results of this decision, we should not forget the message of Judge Lemmon (Felmley, 1981) in the Denver Nurse Inc. case: "The situation is pregnant with the possibility of disrupting the entire economic system of the United States of America." Note Lemmon's choice of words.

CAREER NURSING AND FEMINISM

The career- versus job-orientation dilemma in nursing expresses itself in the ambivalence with which feminist issues have been embraced by career-oriented nurses. With a few notable exceptions, career-oriented nurses have not been seen as sensitive to the rights of women in the health care system. Nursing as a profession has not been in the forefront of recognizing, acknowledging, and creating change in the health care delivery system for women even though most nurses are women.

This has always been of interest to the author because most nurses will also need some type of health care service. Let us examine nursing's past history, beginning with nursing education approximately 20 years ago when it was in its flight from the field of medicine. Nursing curriculums eliminated content specific to the health maintenance of women in favor of a concentration on the maternal role of women. Courses entitled Maternal/Child Health proliferated, and those entitled Obstetrics/Gynecology disappeared. Motherhood is an important female role which represents a significant event, but is nevertheless a limited portion of the lifetime of a woman. This past emphasis in nursing education is reflected in the present difficulty in staffing gynecology clinics and acute care inpatient services for women. Contemporary alternate health care settings for women have had very few nurses involved with their activities.

Career-oriented nurses who are modern-day pioneers in the health care of women are Dr. Anne Burgess of Boston, who has done substantive research and programmatic innovation for victims of rape and sexual assault, and Dr. Ruth Lubic, who is the director of the Maternity Center Association in New York City, an alternative birthing center. These women are to be contrasted to two other (nurse) pioneers who had to reject their attachment to the profession because the nursing role was seen as too limiting or because nursing rejected their work. They are Margaret Sanger, the founder of Planned Parenthood, who only very recently was reclaimed as a hero and placed in Nursing's Hall of Fame; and Wilma Scott Heide, a former president of the National Organization of Women who is presently a Women's Studies professor in the Midwest.

Women's issues and women's health concerns are a primary political event on the national level. Where are career-oriented nurses with respect to these realities? Nurses are becoming more politically sophisticated and active, but are nurses supporting issues related to women's health in addition to those related to other areas of nursing? It is important that efforts to improve the choices for and lives of women not be lost. Such a reversal would have overwhelming implications for all individuals, both females and males. Career nurses can develop their power to bring about a revolution in health care services for women by women.

NURSING EDUCATION AND FEMINISM

Nursing school enrollments in some diploma institutions are increasing. This is not an even national trend in all geographic areas. Associate degree nursing enrollments seem to be increasing too. Nursing education enrollments are, however, dramatically decreasing, particularly in baccalaureate programs in the East. The ability to attract and *retain* bright students in baccalaureate programs is undergoing a metamorphosis. Recently in New York State another private college announced its decision to close its program. In a college publication the following statement was made:

> The problem of the Skidmore Nursing Program is a reflection of the problems existing today within the nursing profession nationally. (*Scope*, 1982)

What is nursing's future? Many career-oriented women are not becoming career-oriented nurses; they are becoming physicians or other professionals where the power dilemma of a career versus a job does not exist.

> Feminism has jolted the profession from two directions, challenging the docility long expected of nurses while simultaneously blasting open other careers for women. At a time when women's roles are being questioned and recast, nursing suffers from less than a glamorous image. Nurses are seen as trafficking in conventionally "female" qualities—compassion, nurturing, and submissiveness. An ambitious woman with a college degree can now opt to enter management, computer science, or the law. (Span, 1980, p. 96)

MEN AND NURSING

Does the entrance of men into the nursing profession improve the career-oriented image? It is difficult for a woman to transgress sex role stereotyping to become a career person. However, in general, she is moving into activities or behaviors valued by the dominant society— male behaviors. Men who enter nursing, on the other hand, are in an extremely difficult position because female nurse behaviors and activities are less valued by society. Therefore, men in nursing are not only transgressing the sex role stereotyping, they are also becoming associated with downwardly mobile female behaviors. Nevertheless, men in nursing achieve leadership positions quickly and in disproportionate numbers within the profession (Hall, 1982). For example in a baccalaureate school of nursing with three types of programs—undergraduate, graduate, and registered nurse (R.N.) track—all of the three student organizations were headed by men, even though their presence in the program was a minimal 27 percent. This can account for the often advanced notion of men as the saviors of nursing—that is, they will create a climate of mutual respect, a higher salary range, and an environment in which nurses can be taken seriously. Men are welcome in nursing, but women in nursing will have to save themselves. Why do female nurses so frequently turn to male nurses to lead them? Can they not see themselves as leaders?

NURSING AND POWER

Another voiced complaint regarding career-oriented nursing deals with the inability of women to work collaboratively with other women. For the large numbers of women who are in nursing, it is significant to note that there are only a very few positions of real power associated with title, status, and money. As in most professions, nurses in powerful positions jealously guard them. There are very few real jobs with power for career-oriented nurses. However, the demand for job-oriented nurses is great. Therefore, competition rather than collaboration results between women in the same profession. The analogy of women on a pedestal applies to career-oriented nursing—there is little room to move about and space is very restricting. Nurses have been on very shaky pedestals. How do nurses come off the pedestal and provide room to nurture their leadership in a more productive and less ''Queen Bee'' fashion? This is an essential question to begin to research because women need to respect other women and must be socialized to do so.

Nursing has been plagued with internal conflicts which can become self-defeating. The women's movement too is presently feeling the pressures of varying approaches: Betty Friedan is advocating a moderate approach to seeking women's rights; while, Sonia Johnson is advocating a continued aggressive approach to seeking women's rights, including those pertaining to reproductive freedom. The internal conflicts that are pervasive in nursing refer to the inability of nurses to recognize, respect, and appreciate the various levels of practice capabilities which exist. Instead, nurses revert to the egalitarian mold within the hospital practice of nursing. Nurses are not all equally competent by virtue of education, commitment, continued learning, experience, and variety of other criteria, but nurses find it difficult to locate appropriate ways to acknowledge and recognize achievement. Nurses need to praise and reward one another to establish power in the health care system. This confusion of values is responsible for a portion of the stress experienced by both the career-oriented nurse and the job-oriented nurse.

The career-oriented nurse, who may be characterized by attributes

such as enthusiasm and assertiveness, needs to be challenged and rewarded. The job-oriented nurse needs to be acknowledged for her contributions, but not placed into roles which require more than she can
give. The job-oriented nurse is frequently content to do her job while
"on duty," but makes a distinct delineation between being "on duty"
and the remainder of her life. The notion of a unification of one's being into a professional person does not exist for her. (This unification
does not imply an inability to put aside the stresses of a job, but does
imply that with a career-oriented nurse the total image and commitment to the profession is not a time-bound function.)

Too often the old practice of seniority in the workplace regulates advancement and access to positions of influence and power. This frequently occurs in hospitals but it is not limited to them. This practice
creates a difficult situation for nursing. The job-oriented nurse finds
herself in positions of leadership about which she may be ambivalent
regarding the responsibility concomitant with the position. Often she
remains in the position, clinging diligently to the status quo, but with
considered respect to her, she delivers the bulk of patient care. The career-oriented nurse seeking to develop herself and the environment for
the delivery of patient care often finds herself frustrated if placed in
the situation of being organizationally responsible to the job-oriented
nurse. In this situation she may elect a number of alternative options,
either outside nursing or within, but usually not in the same work environment.

How does this dilemma in nursing relate to the women's movement?
The author believes the dilemma is a prominent example of the dispar-
ity which exists among women: the conflict of career-orientation versus
job-orientation. The conflict for women is not so much between career
and family, as between a real lifelong career versus limited participation in the workforce. The struggle involves integration of various aspects of life. Women are not uniform or identical in personality or life
style. To require, demand, or seek conformity in women does not make
sense in the wide variety of behaviors exhibited in our heterogeneous
society. Women are seeking the opportunity for all, regardless of gender, to be able to make choices about their lives. Nursing needs to encourage this opportunistic approach more frequently and with more
vigor.

Conformity must no longer be a sacred value in the profession; respect for variety needs to be increased. In the world of practicing nurses
—in the author's opinion—most remain untouched by the women's
movement, a trend which may maximize the more traditional behaviors
of nurses. This trend will continue to influence nursing and its emergence in the 1980s. If nursing cannot solve the dilemma of career- versus

job-orientation, nursing will fill the professional ranks with traditional, conflict-free nurses—powerless persons. Nursing needs women who are powerful career-oriented people.

REFERENCES

Felmley, J. Comparable pay for comparable worth. *Journal of New York State Nurses' Association*, December 1981, *12*(4), 12–16.

Hall, R. Dealing with sexism in nursing and medicine. *Nursing Outlook*, February 1982, *30*(2), 89–94.

McClure, M. Managing the professional nurse. Paper presented at the Journal of Nursing Administration (JONA) Conference, New York City, Spring 1980.

Scope, December 1981–January 1982 (Skidmore College Publication).

Span, P. Where have all the nurses gone? *The New York Times Magazine*, February 22, 1981, pp. 70–101.

[4]

Education

Educating Nurses for Power

Helen M. Lerner

Some say that the nursing profession lacks power. Because of nursing's important role in health care, nurses should be educated to be powerful and effective people. The faculty plays a crucial role in determining how best to educate students to obtain and use power.

Power is a component of all human relationships. Most nurses see themselves as objects of power that other people have and use. Some have assumed attitudes of subordination. These attitudes have contributed to a negative self-image. Nursing education has done little to combat this image problem. For the most part, it has not stimulated self-assertive behavior by the student. The service orientation is still prevalent in nursing programs and this does not equip nurses to project themselves as significant health professionals who can establish power in the health care system. Autonomy, aggression, and competition are rewarded by society. These attributes lead to power and the ability to create and promote changes in society. These attributes have not been fostered enough in nursing education.

Due to nursing's long history of education controlled by hospitals, nursing has allowed others to try to set standards for their practice. If nurses were powerless to set their own standards of practice, they could not perceive themselves as having power in relationship to other professionals within the health care system. Nursing education should be aware of this history and the influence it has upon the issues of rights and power.

There are several issues involved in socializing nursing students to see themselves as persons with power. The following is a description of some of the significant ones.

The first issue is a fundamental one—nursing image. What the public thinks nursing is and how nursing is practiced will influence who chooses nursing as a career, and thus profoundly affect student recruitment. Obviously, the kind of image nurses are given in the media and in society is going to attract a certain group of people to become nurses. To further complicate matters, nursing has changed a great deal over the past 20 years and it always takes a society a long time to begin to incorporate these changes. The public is often unaware of developments taking place within the nursing profession and the range of services the nurse has to offer.

Television is the most influential information medium in our society. Many opinions held by the public are derived from the image of nurses seen on television. In a study done by Kalisch and Kalisch (1982) nurses on television were depicted as the handmaidens of the physician or used as background scenery for hospital dramas. They found in a content analysis of personal attributes that physicians on television demonstrated higher levels of ambition, intelligence, risk taking, adeptness, self-confidence, and sophistication than did nurses. They even were noted to show higher levels of sincerity, altruism, and honesty than were nurses, in spite of the fact that these latter values have often been attributed to nurses. Nurses scored high on obedience, permissiveness, conformity, and flexibility.

If nurses are consistently represented this way on television, students who are recruited into the profession will already have assimilated this negative stereotype. Nursing cannot have high prestige as a career if it is consistently devalued in the media. It is also going to be difficult for nurses to command respect as knowledgeable professionals if the public is constantly exposed to a negative image of nursing.

Persons of high economic status have not traditionally directed their children toward nursing. Some nursing students are from middle or lower socioeconomic groups. These groups have not traditionally had power within society. The problem of nursing image and a student body that comprises primarily women from middle or lower socioeconomic status presents problems in recruiting students who expect to use power.

But the outlook for changing nursing's image and recruitment into the profession is not as bleak as it appears. If the image of nursing is changing slowly, the image of women is undergoing a more rapid change. The women's liberation movement and the effect that it has had on society have begun to help the nursing profession. True, it has opened up more careers to women so that there is more competition for potential nursing students. Yet, it has also helped to bring nursing economic issues such as salaries, chauvinistic treatment, and poor working conditions into the open because they are closely tied with women's economic issues. The women's movement is forcing the public to pay attention to these issues.

Moving nursing education onto the college campuses has exposed nursing students to campus activism, protest, and organizations which are trying to affect change. Nursing faculty should encourage participation in these groups during the nursing program so that students learn first-hand about power and how to facilitate change.

In addition, high school guidance counselors must constantly be brought up to date on the changes in nursing. They must be helped to present nursing as a serious career for intelligent women. The profession must not be viewed as temporary employment or a good job for a woman going back to work.

The second issue is the education of students to recognize the value of the autonomous function of nursing. Nursing stands by itself in its contribution to both care and cure. It is often nursing alone that makes the difference to a patient. This should be pointed out to students as part of their own clinical practice and nursing practice in general. Autonomous nursing actions that do not require or relate to physician's direction change outcomes for patients.

The following clinical situation illustrates this point. A young primipara entered the hospital in early labor. She was three to four centimeters dilated and was having difficulty coping with contractions even though she had gone to prepared childbirth classes. The patient's husband was present. There was considerable friction between the couple. The husband felt that if his wife did not want to "go through with it" she had wasted their time attending the classes. The physicians were reluctantly preparing to give the patient a rather large dose of sedation which could have proved dangerous to her labor. The nursing student stood listening to the physician. The instructor suggested that what was needed here was not pharmacological intervention, but nursing care.

The student went in to stay with the patient. She took the husband aside and suggested he relax, take a short break, go for coffee. She demonstrated breathing techniques to the patient with each contraction and with some effort had the patient working with her. When the husband returned from coffee, the student gradually let him assume the coaching role. A few minutes later the physician entered the room to tell the patient she could have her medication now. The patient replied, "I don't need it." The labor progressed normally, and both husband and wife reported a very satisfactory labor experience.

The student did for the patient what only a nurse could do. Her knowledge gave her power over the situation and changed the outcome for the patient. With enough of these experiences, students can begin to integrate the fact that they alone can make the difference for a patient and family.

The third issue involving power in nursing is unity in the profession. Faculty members can be role models in this area. Efforts can be made to bridge the gap between service and education. Time should not be spent discussing the shortcomings of each. Students need to understand and respect all nurses. (Faculty need to encourage students to seek the expertise of staff nurses.) The faculty themselves should make efforts to share their research with nurses in the clinical settings and share ideas about patient care. Not all nursing actions seen are laudable, but there are many that are. Nurses need to focus on these and give students a viable group of role models with which to identify. A unified group can certainly exert power more effectively.

By helping students identify themselves as part of nursing, these students are helped to find a basis for relationships with other health professionals. Nursing has had difficulty differentiating itself from medicine. The relationship of nursing and medicine takes the form of a patriarchal power structure in a world where masculine attributes are more highly valued than are feminine attributes. Rodgers (1981) states that professionals who exert the greatest leadership are those whose professional identity is secure and who have a genuine tolerance of ambiguity. Nursing has difficulty negotiating psychological separation from medicine. Successful separation and individuation will result in the profession's assumption of responsibility for nursing care and less of an intense need to defend themselves. Nursing students should learn to relate to physicians in ways that recognize the value of both professions. They need learning experiences with medical students that will sensitize both groups to the needs of one another and the contribution that each makes to the care of the patient and family. Difficulties in nurse-physician relationships should be dealt with in a constructive manner, not in a passive-aggressive way which only perpetuates the conflict. Nursing faculty need to become role models for students in resolving these kinds of conflicts constructively. Nurses who respect one another and who can relate with other professionals in a positive and assertive way can become a group which can exert a formidable source of power.

The fourth issue is, nursing students need to realize that knowledge is power. They need to feel competent as nurses and to know that they are held to a standard of excellence.

Clinical experiences for students that will build their feelings of confidence must be provided. Confidence is not developed in observational situations. The kind of experiences that permit involvement in actual care promote development of both technical and interpersonal skills and encourage thinking. These experiences allow students to take responsibility for their own actions. Davidhizor (1982) thinks the instructor should be a supportive facilitator in the situation and enable the students to decide on their own course of action. A powerful person is one who is knowledgeable and self-confident.

From the beginning, the faculty should emphasize that nursing is an intellectual discipline as well as a practical one. Knowledge is an essential component of power. Faculty should share their research with students from the beginning of the program.

Cleland (1971) states that the traditional preparation of nurses included dependency characteristics and predictable behaviors. Thus, nurses tend to respond to predictable situations and ask others about unpredictable ones. Students should be prepared to think and plan for the unpredictable. Mahoney (1980) found that many senior students in baccalaureate nursing programs seemed unsure of their roles or were unable to deal with a complex client situation in which multiple problems existed; data were incomplete and hypotheses rather than knowns were needed to guide their actions. Professional nurses are expected to deal with various abstractions, complexities, and situations that are not clearly defined. If nurses can do this they will not rely so much on the direction of others such as physicians and hospital administrators.

If we pursue these policies in nursing educational programs, nursing can hope to begin to produce nurses who can obtain and exercise power for their own and nursing's future.

REFERENCES

Cleland, V. Sex discrimination: Nursing's most pervasive problem. *American Journal of Nursing*, 1971, *71*, 1542–1547.

Davidhizor, R. Helping students to help themselves. *Nursing and Health Care*, 1982, *3*, 138–142.

Kalisch, P. A., & Kalisch, B. J. Nurses on prime time television. *American Journal of Nursing*, 1982, *82*, 264–270.

Mahoney, A. Decision making by senior students in baccalaureate nursing

programs. Unpublished doctoral dissertation, Teachers College, Columbia University, 1980.
Rodgers, J. A. Toward professional adulthood. *Nursing Outlook*, 1981, *29*, 478–
481.

Nursing and Internal Politics: A View from the Periphery Based on Personal Experience

Lois G. Muzio

INTRODUCTION

When nurses think of political power, they are likely to see it primarily in relation to struggles with forces outside of the nursing community. Nurses have the ability to protect their territory from external incursions and controls, to promote their interests through competition and in cooperation with other interest groups within the health care system, and to secure for themselves at least a fair share of that system's benefits. Certainly, the positive political training that resulted from the turbulent 1960s across this country coupled with the women's rights movement in recent years have been major contributory factors to our awareness.

Nurses should applaud the efforts of nursing professional organizations and lobby groups which influence changes in health policy, legislation, and funding that support the profession. When political endeavors succeed, nurses interpret the event as a signal of the maturing of the profession. However, political power is a tool that can be directed toward those within the profession as well as toward those external to it.

The purpose of this chapter is to offer a caveat on the use of political power in nursing education. The internal exercise of political power can control and promote the direction of change according to agreed-upon goals. It can also be effectively used to prevent change, to protect those in power, and—by impeding access to education, credentials, or jobs—it can exclude certain constituencies. When employed in this negative manner, existing patterns of practice and education, as well as their supporting structures, can be protected from the threat of competition. To some—usually those who would benefit from controlling the direction of or preventing change—sustaining the status quo is obviously beneficial. To others, it seems not unlike the reactionary and protectionist responses of the already familiar power groups in the health care system. Apparently, it is far easier to call for changes in other professional groups than it is to accept and/or promote internal calls for change that vary from the prevalent ideas of the majority.

In nursing education, the political in-group represents traditional, well-established educational programs, along with the various associations and policy-making bodies that are designed to aid, support, and perpetuate these programs. The political out-group consists of those who are not associated with these traditional educational structures: those who would oppose, alter, or offer alternatives to traditional nursing education. Over time, the out-group membership has changed. Those who sought to establish associate degree programs were one-time members; the developers of the recent Regent's External Degree Program were members, and to a certain extent may still be; the proponents of a career-ladder and other nontraditional approaches are still under scrutiny by the educational "middle-of-the-roaders." And even further out on the periphery are those who would provide for the evaluation and granting of college credit for experiential learning, or construct individualized nursing programs for some of the registered nurse population.

The tendency to resist, impede, or oppose innovative efforts—almost as if they were produced by external forces to threaten the very course of the profession—is an understandable but potentially harmful response of the political in-group members. Such use of political power can effectively exclude the serious and needed consideration of possibly good ideas that address current issues and problems, that respond sensitively to changing times and conditions, and that require further experimentation in the open forum of educational research.

The experience of conducting a feasibility study for an experimental nontraditional BSN program for registered nurses at Empire State College, State University of New York (SUNY) demonstrated to the author how effectively nurses in powerful positions can protect their own territories from competition, however small it may be. Clearly, there are and should be legitimate and substantive questions regarding any new educational proposals. This is a vital part of the developmental process.

But, opposition without regard to the quality of the proposal or the needs of the constituents to be served—purely for the purpose of protecting existing programs and structures—is something entirely different.

One of the major problems for the innovator in nursing education has become the high cost of counteracting the opposition from within the nursing community. The initiation of a new program may not be worth the economic costs. For example, it is estimated that the New York State Regent's External Degree Program spent at least $180,000 to overcome opposition to its BSN program and to achieve accreditation. The preparation of innumerable reports, appearances at many hearings, legal costs, administrative costs, and the appeal processes were expensive and energy-wasting experiences. It should be noted that the establishment of a new but traditional program certainly would never have involved comparable economic and human energy expenditures.

Although the final act has not been written, it now appears that Empire State College (SUNY) will not proceed with its proposed experimental program for registered nurses at this time, even though there is a large constituency for such a program, and despite the proposed legislation that would support programs designed to meet the needs of registered nurses. It is patently clear that the high cost of offsetting the opposition within the nursing community is a main concern that has led to the reconsideration of the Empire State College proposal. Such costs would possibly hamper other nontraditional program proposals in the future.

Is it possible that growth in the ability to use political power on behalf of all of nursing has as its intrinsic concomitant the ability to resist internal change? If so, then the future will certainly be one of less flexibility, less diversity, and less growth. While these comments may appear to be a polemic to some readers, it is hoped that awareness of such possibilities could lead to refinements in the uses of power. New approaches in nursing education need open discussion, sound experimentation, and evaluation as integral parts of the consideration process. New program proposals should be considered as educational research and not viewed as simply threats to existing political power bases.

Reaching for Power from Within

Ann Costello Galligan

INTRODUCTION

Few would dispute that many of the problems inherent in the nursing profession to date have been a direct result of the stereotype of women in general. Historically, women were socialized to be self-sacrificing for mother, father, brother, husband, and children. They learned early that to subordinate their needs for the sake of others resulted in the least amount of opposition and the highest degree of acceptance. Moreover, assertiveness—which was more than likely perceived as aggression— was deemed to be a not-so-ladylike characteristic.

Women have been socialized in the past to view power and independence as negative characteristics. While most men have viewed their career as a lifelong pursuit leading upward with rewards, increases in salary, recognition, and status, few women have regarded their careers as a lifelong pursuit. Women in their middle years were not encouraged to take careers or professional goals seriously while planning for them in young adulthood. Those that did were often too soon discouraged by both their immediate social surroundings (i.e., family, friends) and the larger social system (i.e., religious organizations, cultural affiliations). Ultimately, the stress arising from these powerful influences was traumatic enough to affect even the most self-confident of women. Understandably, the role of the dependent victim had become a more appropriate ploy to achieve an effective end.

The suffragist movement and the more recent women's movement originating in the 1960s provoked a conscious awareness that equality and autonomy for women were inherent rights, not privileges. Unfortunately, while the leaders in the feminist movement have made this vision a reality, most women persist in feeling "guilty" for pursuing personal and professional goals. More bewildering is the fact that, despite the plethora of choices available today, there persists a sense of powerlessness among women toward the achievement of goals. Thus in the eighth decade of the twentieth century, women continue to perceive themselves and their careers as less significant than those of their male counterparts.

The nursing profession has been slow to internalize the feminists' underlying message of self-determination and commitment. Historically, nurses have looked upon their contribution as a temporary stepping stone until something better came along, usually an improved economic situation achieved through marriage or a spouse's professional advancement. Nursing was believed by some women to be "a job you did" to supplement a deficient economic situation or to afford that something extra (for example, a new washing machine, family vacation). Of course, once the financial situation was rectified, the nurse was expected to resign to attend to her family commitments until some future date when her job income would be needed again.

Parallelling the women's role in the larger society, nursing has perceived itself as the victim of the health care system. Nursing salaries and benefits have not been pressing issues on hospital boards because it was assumed that the nurses (women) were not the principal breadwinners of the family. Furthermore, selected benefits (retirement, medical, and dental plans) have been ignored, since it was believed that they were subsumed elsewhere (for example, in the spouse's plan). Rather than question or dispute the basis for these discriminations as most men might, nurses reverted to their role as victim and accepted their dilemma. Nurses have perceived themselves as "objects of the power of others and have tended to internalize the attitudes of subordination projected by those in authority and by other health professionals" (Brooten, Mayman, & Naylor, 1978, p. 56).

Nursing is perhaps the only profession whose membership consists almost entirely of women—over one million of them. If strength is equated with numbers, why then has the profession experienced such difficulty in channeling its strength to achieve status, recognition, and power? It may be that women have not fully internalized the necessity for a long-term professional commitment, which not only enhances personal growth but also strengthens the profession from within. Just as children need nurturance to attain their maximum potential, so does the profession of nursing—if it is to mature beyond its internal structure and function. With a firm commitment of its members, nursing will grow to its maximum potential, expand its boundaries, and ultimately contribute to the growth of other professions and society at large.

How then does nursing achieve a firm commitment from its membership? It is this author's contention that the two most salient characteristics associated with the long-term commitment to any profession are one's self-esteem and perception of power. As educators, it may be wise to nurture these qualities in students from the outset of their educational programs if nursing is to enhance their growth and development.

Kanter (1981) has defined power as "the capacity to mobilize people and get things done." Moreover, personal strength, which is the most important element in the personal power base, is derived from a strong and realistic self-concept. Thus, power is accomplished through capacity or efficacy, rather than domination or control. People who lack power, or, more tragically, perceive themselves as powerless, are often less effective. Just as crab grass can quickly infiltrate and cause damage to an entire lawn and those nearby, so too can a sense of powerlessness spread throughout an entire organization and its related systems.

Coopersmith (1967, p. 12) defines self-esteem as "the extent to which the individual believes himself to be capable, significant, successful, and worthy." Subsequently, the more worthy a person regards himself to be, the more likely he will adapt a more active and assertive position. Coopersmith contends that two of the factors contributing to an individual's self-esteem are his acceptance by significant others and his history of successes within his frame of reference. Self-esteem has not been evident in recent nursing students or recent baccalaureate graduates. Moreover, one only has to listen to nursing's more experienced practitioners to realize that self-esteem has neither been developed nor acquired over time.

Although the sense of powerlessness, evident in nursing today, is epidemic, it is not a new phenomenon to the profession. Nurses, and women in general, have always felt powerless. However, the phenomenon that has provoked an all-time low morale within the professional membership has been a noticeable lack in self-esteem which appears to be universal. In view of this latter fact, one has to ask the question, why?

Until the late 1960s and early 1970s, women as well as men had a strong concept of gender identity. Right or wrong, good or bad, women were in little conflict with their role in society. Nursing was an admired profession despite its many limitations. Students of nursing learned early that they were the "best" and those fortunate enough to be graduates of a baccalaureate program knew well that they were considered the "elite." Expectations were high for these graduates, and there was no doubt that they would make a significant contribution to the profession.

The women's movement made us aware of women's rights to autonomy and power and the values inherent therein. Since the underlying message of the women's movement was to strive for equality and self-fulfillment, women began choosing more diverse careers than ever before. Moreover, male-dominated professions such as business, law, and medicine were soon being well-represented by women.

Unfortunately for some, this restructuring of societal norms provoked conflict within the profession of nursing since it led to the misconception that "male" was better. Students, who may have once chosen nursing, selected other professions such as medicine because it was deemed significantly a better choice. Some left nursing for another career. It appears that many were deeply affected by the prevailing non-accepting attitude of other professionals and larger society. Moreover, because nurses began questioning their own sense of worth, it was easy to understand why others external to the profession did as well.

Those remaining "loyal" to nursing as a profession have not only experienced an overwhelming sense of powerlessness but have also been stripped of their own sense of self-esteem. This was once an innate strength of the profession. An ameliorated sense of self-esteem has hampered efforts for assertiveness and change by its membership which are necessary for nursing survival today.

Nursing faculty is responsible for affecting a sense of power within the nursing educational system. More specifically, nursing faculty need to develop an awareness among students of their potential ability to effect change. The women's movement has given nurses the impetus to strive for power and change. Therefore, nursing faculty must work diligently to reframe the negativity that is rampant within the profession toward a more positive attitude. This is not an easy task since men have always had the power. As Jessie Bernard (Abrams, 1981) suggests, it may be necessary to make "pests" of ourselves for a time in order to disturb the normal rhythm of things. This is necessary since no individual with power will give it away willingly (Abrams, 1981).

At the outset, faculty must strive to enhance self-esteem and a strong self-concept among students. Basically, nurse educators must begin working from within the educational system so as to develop a positive energy field and a strong sense of commitment toward the profession. Just as graduates of business and medical schools are taught early that they are the "elite," nursing faculty must plant the seed in each student's mind that they too are the "elite." Moreover, it is important that students know from the beginning that they are members of one of the oldest surviving professions, founded and strengthened by women. It is important that students understand that they are expected to continue the tradition and make a significant contribution to society. Hopefully, faculty can discourage students from thinking of themselves as powerless and encourage them to make a lifelong commitment to the nursing profession.

It is paramount that nurse educators begin working from within the educational system so as to develop a positive energy field. If this energy can be channeled appropriately, a more positive attitude will prevail which will eventually infiltrate the larger health care industry. Students must not only be aware of their particular role within the nursing profession, but they must be aware also of their role in relation to the larger political system of which they are a part. To do this students need to be encouraged, early, to be creative thinkers, to question the norm, to voice opinions, and to recognize the choices that are available to them. They must be encouraged to be change agents, leaders, decision makers, and "heads" of systems, rather than passive participants. Only then will nursing attain the status and prestige it once held.

REFERENCES

Abrams, M. The woman's world of Jessie Bernard. *Graduate Woman*, 1981, *75*(4), 26.

Brooten, D., Mayman, L., & Naylor, M. *Leadership for change: A guide for the frustrated nurse*. New York: J. B. Lippincott Company, 1978.

Coopersmith, S. *The antecedents of self-esteem*. San Francisco: W. H. Freeman and Company, 1967.

Kanter, R. Leadership for the twenty-first century. *Theory into Practice*, 1981, *20*(4), 221.

Professional Nursing Associations

Power and the Professional Association

Lucille A. Joel

The single most powerful instrument available to nurses is the professional association. By design, the professional association safeguards the autonomy of practice by establishing standards for assessing the quality of service and for monitoring the ranks of practitioners. Without this self-determination there is no professional pride. There is no sense of the basic decency and utility of one's work.

Though this reasoning is moving, it lacks credibility unless it is logically justified. The case for the role and function of professional associations derives from the basic nature of society's charge to the professions. Professions come into existence and are sustained when they are needed for a unique service. In what should be a mutually enriching relationship, the consumer recognizes the prescriptive ability of the practitioner and professionals remain sensitive to evolving social requirements. Though human needs remain relatively stable, the context for the delivery of services does not. New workers enter the health care scene; technology changes; new settings for service prove themselves; and so on. There is an ever-present obligation to redefine a profession's scope and entry requirements for practice. These are central policy decisions which, for the sake of credibility, must be made by incumbents of the profession. Wisdom dictates that nurses carefully listen to our communities of interest, but prudence warns that the right to decide must be jealously guarded by the profession. Professional associations provide the arena for this decision making. It would be inappropriate to have these policies evolve from regulatory agencies with obvious consumer biases or groups which allow lay membership. Once these decisions slip from our grasp, our autonomy will quickly erode. Power lies in nurses defining nursing practice for nurses.

Before nurses had any great sense that there would ever be a need to safeguard their territorial prerogatives, some visionary and pioneering leaders assured the practice domain of nursing through an individual licensing act. This model is usual among professionals. The license becomes personal property, and so the individual's commitment to the service weighs more heavily than commitment to any institution or employer. The entrepreneurial nature of professions has created a healthy respect for collective strength through professional societies or associations. Individual responsibility can result in the watering down of quality unless there is some objective practice standard promulgated by the profession itself. History is rich with evidence that the professions are expected to provide internal control over both service and providers. Even where pieces of this responsibility fall to governmental regulatory agencies, the policies promulgated by the profession should continue to provide a basis for action. Nurses as salaried professionals are atypical and have been slow to recognize the nature of their license, the need for networking their human resources, and the need to speak with one voice.

Throughout its history, the American Nurses' Association has grown to a fuller appreciation of its role as nursing has grown to fuller status as a profession. The Association came to grips with policy decisions concerning scope, standards, and credentialing at a point when few incumbents of the profession realized the need for these documents. Though associational leadership has labored under a constant barrage of internal conflict and criticism, it held to a firm course toward an agenda which would begin to establish our status as a profession. The American Nurses' Association has made progress despite the fact that only 10 percent of practicing nurses are members. In their naivete, nurses have been lulled into complacency. The power of their numbers has been hidden from their awareness. Nurses are burdened by the day-to-day demands of work, and have never been socialized to expect professional control of their practice—but this has not been a central concern. Ironically, our practice acts give us more latitude to function than nurses have dared to use. An appreciation of these prerogatives brings new awareness of the need to support the work of the American Nurses' Association.

Power in politics and policy making requires careful orchestration of resources on the local, state, and federal scene. There is a new appreciation of the way ineffectiveness at any one level weakens the entire system. Recent debate over the most adequate structure for the American Nurses' Association has gotten past the what-can-you-do-for-me mentality, and onto the question of how we can increase our collective strength through synchronizing our activities more carefully. There is a new and growing need to network within the profession, to speak out on issues, and to have a strong national associational voice for nursing. A recent flurry of activity to organize nurses for a variety of purposes, including collective bargaining, continuing education, and single issue militancy threatens to fragment our numbers. The American Nurses' Association will only speak for nursing as long as it represents more nurses than any other organization. Our representativeness is already being challenged. It becomes difficult to influence public policy and cultivate political alliances when the organization can no longer claim to speak for large numbers of individuals and consequently the profession. As these ideas take shape, association policies and programs become more palatable as either an end in themselves or as a means to an end. Programs which draw membership become essential. If wage and salary issues and collective bargaining services are necessary for the welfare of a large number of nurses, organized nursing has no option but to offer these programs.

In summary, the mission of the professional association is to tend to the care and feeding of the profession. The power to address this charge and to be influential in policy making and political arenas derives from control of practice. Control of practice can be reduced to two basic elements: service and provider. The professional association assumes the responsibility to define standards for quality care, and establish the qualifications for entry into the profession as well as criteria for specialty practice. Despite our right to speak, we will never be heard unless our membership base is maintained and grows.

Nursing, Policy, and the Association

Cathryne A. Welch

INTRODUCTION

Health policy affects nursing practice, education, research, and administration. Therefore, it is a logical assumption that nurses are involved in establishing health policy, implementing health policy, and making health policy decisions. In order to pursue the truth of the assumption, the author turned to the usual sources of information about health policy research in the nursing literature. The following facts were established:

• *Cumulative Index to Nursing and Allied Health Literature* yielded references on health policy (Cumulative Index, 1956–1982).
• *Nursing Studies Index* 1900–1959 yielded no references on health policy (Nursing Studies, 1963–1972).
• *International Nursing Index* yielded no references until 1980. Those health policy research studies which do appear post-1980 are primarily interrogations, assertions, and admonitions about policy. Research studies on health policy with sound methodology are absent (International Nursing, 1969–1983).
• *Nursing III, A Selected Collection of Academic and Professional Research Materials* yielded studies under the heading of policy through 1980 (Nursing III, 1980).

Health policy research in the nursing literature is scant, so the author decided to seek immediate refuge in the standard dictionary references. The term *policy* was researched through this vehicle. The following information was found:

• *Brittanica World Language Dictionary* (1980) defines policy as (1) prudence or sagacity in the conduct of affairs; (2) a course or plan of action, especially of administrative action; (3) any system of management based on self-interest as opposed to equity; finesse in general; artifice; (4) Obsolete—political science, government; (5) a written contract of insurance; (6) a gambling game.

- *Black's Law Dictionary* defined policy as the general principles by which a government is guided in its management of public affairs, or the legislature in its measures. Public policy was defined as that principle of law which holds that no subject can lawfully do that which has a tendency to be injurious to the public or against the public good (Black, 1979).
- *Oxford American Dictionary, 1980* defined policy as the course or general plan of action adopted by a government or party or person (Ehrlich, 1980).
- *Random House Dictionary, 1978* defined policy as (1) a guiding principle or course of action adopted toward an objective or objectives; (2) prudence or practical wisdom (Stein, 1978).

Finally it was clear to the author that not only was research on the topic scarce but also dictionaries were not very helpful. A decision was then made to focus on the author's own ideas about nursing and health policy.

NURSING POLICY

The nursing profession has clearly and repeatedly enunciated its policy on health. Since the birth of organized nursing that policy has been to further the efficient care of the sick and disabled and others in need of nursing services. Essential to fulfillment of policy have been (1) the development of and maintenance of proper standards—of nursing education and practice; and (2) insurance of an adequate supply of qualified nurses. Throughout nursing's history, our policy on health has been unrestricted by consideration of race, creed, color, or socioeconomic status.

Formulation of health policy has long been a goal. As a profession, nursing has not been a major determinant of health policy in this country. Nursing has been instead shaped and molded by the social and economic forces of the times. Predominantly, nursing has been in a reactionary or responsive state versus the creative role with respect to designing health policy. Frankly, the author believes that nursing has stood on the periphery of both power and politics for so long as a result of its inability to use its own force in the formulation of health policy.

The author further believes that the profession now stands at the brink of opportunity as a result of what is the most dramatic social trend of the 1980s: a shift toward the value of individualism.

Toward Individualism

The United States of America has progressed substantially in the direction of the socialized or welfare state. However, recent national elections suggest a significant number of Americans wish to curtail, if not reverse, this direction. This shift should not come as a surprise. For some years social, economic, and political analysts have warned of the debilitating impact that increased institutionalization on society would have on people. Roche's summary is representative of this point of view:

> Today, the typical American finds himself confronted with "bigness" on an unprecedented scale. Our lives are institutionalized and regulated on every hand. Each of us is becoming a smaller and smaller chip floating on a more and more enormous ocean. The individual finds himself under great pressure from every quarter to "adjust" . . . to find a place in "the system."
>
> Since all the institutions of our society make the same demand, the individual has no place to turn. . . . On every hand he meets a denial that the individual is genuinely significant; on every hand he is confronted with vast institutional enmassments that seem beyond both his control and comprehension. . . . Self-determination seems to be leaving us—the world grows larger and larger, our institutions grow larger; and in the process there seems less self-determination for individuals and a constantly growing role for big business, big labor, big education, big Foundations, big TV networks, and above all—big government. (Roche, 1981, p. 1)

Americans have blown the whistle on the trend toward institutionalization.

The political and economic consequences of these actions are quite profound. Indeed, stunning political defeats and victories have occurred; still others are threatened or promised, depending on one's perspective. The magnitude of the economic impact in the country is illustrated by the "employing" and "expending" characteristics of government:

> In 1940 all American governments—Federal, state, and local—were employing 4,474,000 people. In 1977, the number was 14,624,000. The Federal government alone, in 1978, employed 2,066,000 persons in its armed forces and 1,930,100 in full-time permanent civilian employment. In addition, it

was making Social Security payments to some 33 million persons and the Congressional Budget office was estimating that about 44 million were receiving some sort of welfare aid.

The annual expenditures of the federal government tell a succinct story. If we take them at ten-year intervals since 1929, we get the following result:

Year	Expenditures	
1929	$3.1 billion	
1939	8.8 billion	
1949	38.8 billion	
1959	92.1 billion	
1969	184.5 billion	
1979	487.5 billion	(Hazlitt, 1979)

The United States may stand at the threshold of a major dismantling of society's systems, institutions, agencies, programs, and policies.

However, daily media reports inform the people that "the system" and its diverse advocates and beneficiaries will not "go gently unto that good night." The land abounds with coalitions, task forces, and motley get-togethers forging strategies and methodologies to preserve at least some portion of their share of governmental largesse.

Nursing is part of this scramble. As a profession it has precious little to lose and it must guard its relatively meager societal support with particular vigilance and skill. Nursing should raise its collective professional voice now in support of health programs which should legitimately be financed by government.

Opportunities for Nursing

The author will not comment on the possible or probable roles and influence of special interest lobbies versus the citizenry-at-large. Nor will the author dwell on those current programs the nursing profession should support or renounce. Instead, this paper will identify three dimensions of the shift toward individualism which are consistent with the nature and responsibilities of nursing and which offer the nursing profession desperately needed opportunities for implementing its policy.

People want, need, and are seeking not simply health care, but humanized health care. The phrase humanized health care seems on its face redundant. Indeed, there have been attempts to increase access to health care for more and more people, but the care itself has frequently been fragmented and discontinuous, lacking compassion as well as coordination.

Rising public interest in and understanding of health care is well-documented. So too is readiness for participation in decision making about the nature of health care to be rendered, the settings in which health care ought to be available, and the matrix of significant others/family and prepared personnel who will act as providers. The public is now demonstrating impatience with aspects of institutionalized health care which the nursing profession for far too long has been either willing to accept or unable to change.

In December 1980, the American Nurses' Association (in "Nursing: A Social Policy Statement") reminded nurses and others of these nursing verities:

> Nurses are guided by a humanistic philosophy, having care coupled with understanding and purpose as its central feature. Nurses have the highest regard for self-determination, independence, and choice in decision making in matters of health.

> Nurses are committed to respecting human beings because of a profound regard for humanity. This principle applies to themselves, to people receiving care, and to other people who share in the provision of care.

> Nursing care is provided in an interpersonal relationship process of nurse-with-a-patient, nurse-with-a-family, nurse-with-a-group. It involves privileged intimacy—physical and interpersonal.

Yet the nursing profession has not, to any significant extent, unshackled itself from either the physician-handmaiden or institutional lackey role. Nursing licensure contracts have been with patients, but in the main, the profession's loyalties have been elsewhere. One knows fine nursing practice does go on—but one has but to be hospitalized—or to worry through the hospitalization of a loved one—to witness the alarming abdication of nursing responsibilities by far too many so-called professional nurses. Perhaps the revival of individualism and the renewal of interest in self-determination will give nurses the courage to stand for patients and ourselves.

Declining confidence in and dependence on government can enhance the nursing profession's legitimate self-determination and self-regulation activities. As government has grown in this country, it has become fashionable to attribute a sinister self-interest to all activities, organizations, and agencies existing outside the governmental sphere. Where no tangible evidence of such could be found, potential interest conflict justified governmental intrusion in the activities and processes previously of an essentially voluntary nature.

Business and industry have loudly expressed their disenchantment with a kind and degree of regulation that stifle. Even the sacred professions whose very existence generates from a social contract based on grants of public trust and authority have been drawn into the web of heightened governmental surveillance and subjugation. Thus, this country has witnessed mandates for consumer involvement in a host of professional regulatory activities and concomitant prohibitions against expression by professions of their legitimate needs, expertise, and prerogatives.

Certain health care groups—notably the medical profession and hospital industry—have resisted, sometimes through litigation, those laws, rules, and regulations they deem unduly oppressive or inimical to public interest. Nursing, however, has generally quietly acquiesced.

State Boards for Nursing have systematically distanced themselves from the profession. Their composition swells with more and more public representatives. The administrative agencies in which these boards are housed offer ever-increasing challenges to the professional organization's involvement in the development and implementation of policy, laws, rules, and regulations impacting on nursing and health care. Educational initiatives, long the subject of verbal endorsement by the profession, have languished in the face of ill-informed allegations of restriction of goods and services or cartel development. And the American Nurses' Association itself has recently supported the establishing of a freestanding credentialing center which presumably, through some ambiguous consultative process with sundry groups, will offer greater public protection than the profession itself can (or should the author say, is willing to?) guarantee. Perhaps the diminution of governmental influence will rekindle the profession's enthusiasm for self-regulation and restore its confidence in its ability to assume this vital professional obligation.

The breakup and/or breakdown of existing systems can permit and encourage increased autonomy and creativity in nursing practice. For decades nurses have practiced predominantly as employees. In this context, the barriers to implementation of legal responsibilities to patients have been enormous. Furthermore, lack of understanding and respect for nursing practice and practitioners by employers and other health care providers have perpetuated deplorable employment conditions. As countless workers throughout history have done—including most notably the Polish Solidarity—nurses turned to collective bargaining as a means of exercising and protecting their lawful responsibilities and rights.

The vast majority of nurses who elected to use this instrument of self-actualization turned to the professional society for assistance. Hence, state nurses associations are the major representatives of registered professional nurses in this country. This was no easy achievement, for there has been within many segments of the nursing community a challenging, grudging, and/or condescending attitude toward collective bargaining. It has been perceived alternately as unnecessary, unprofessional, or undesirable, but nonetheless it is a necessary tool for the unfortunate or handicapped within the profession. The author calls particular attention to the latter because it is so representative of one of nursing's major developmental weaknesses as a profession: Nurses themselves have not accepted the tremendous responsibility, worth, and dignity of their own nursing practice. In their failure to do so, nurses have undervalued the practitioner and almost unconsciously relegated the "staff nurse" to an implied underlying and undeserving position.

The profession is rapidly being jolted out of this stage of development. Other labor organizations confronted with declining memberships, declining population, and declining worker interest are searching frantically for new constituencies and power bases. Although nurses have not always been aware of it, nursing is hard to miss! As the leader of one competing labor organization has observed: "The population is declining, but living longer. Jobs for others will dry up, but not for nurses. Health service and nurses will be in greater and greater demand. The organization that represents nurses will be around a lot longer than the organization for whom the labor market is disappearing." Indirectly, the massive assault by competing labor organizations has alerted us to the essential nature of the profession's services and accountability for those services.

Obviously, the profession must and can retain its control over collective bargaining for professional nurses. Prior to the Depression, nursing practice was largely entrepreneurial. The shift toward individualism together with efforts to control costs and reduce waste and corruption in health care will prompt creation of some new and some old practice modes, settings, and patterns. Perhaps these trends will reawaken nursing's pioneer spirit and lead to a reduction in reliance on and practice through the employee role.

SUMMARY

Each of the opportunities identified for nursing have begun in sentences beginning with the word "perhaps."

Perhaps the revival of individualism and the renewal of interest in self-determination will give nurses the courage to stand for patients and ourselves.

Perhaps the diminution of governmental influence will rekindle the profession's enthusiasm for and restore its confidence in its ability to assume this vital professional obligation.

Perhaps the shift toward individualism together with efforts to contain costs and reduce waste and corruption in health care will reawaken nursing's pioneer spirit and lead to a reduction in reliance on and practice through the employee role.

The word "perhaps" was chosen not because the author was either pessimistic or cautious—on the contrary, the author is both optimistic and enormously confident. The "perhaps" is meant to emphasize the need for individual nurses to assume responsibility for seizing and acting on the opportunities at hand for implementing nursing policy. If nurses do so, the profession will secure entry requirements, control nurse practice acts, and ensure proper reimbursement for nursing services—and research on the effects of nursing health policy will abound!

REFERENCES

Black, H. C. *Black's Law Dictionary*. (5th ed.) St. Paul, Minn.: West Publishing Company, 1979.

Brittanica World Language Dictionary, 1980.

Cumulative Index to Nursing and Allied Health Literature. (Vols. 1–27). Glendale, Calif.: Glendale Adventist Medical Center, 1956–1982.

Ehrlich, E., Flexner, S. B., Carruth, G., & Hawkins, J. M. *Oxford American Dictionary*. New York: Avon Books, 1980.

Hazlitt, H. The torrents of laws. *The Freeman* (Foundation for Economic Development, Irvington-on-Hudson, New York), January 1979, *29*, 10.

International Nursing Index. (Vols. 1–17). New York: American Journal of Nursing Company, 1969–1983.

Nursing: A Social Policy Statement. Publication Code No. NP–63–35M. Kansas City, Mo.: American Nurses' Association, 1980.

Nursing III, A Selected Collection of Academic and Professional Research Materials. Ann Arbor, Mich.: University Microfilms International, 1980.

Nursing Studies Index. (Vols. I–IV, 1900–1959). Philadelphia: J. B. Lippincott, 1963–1972.

Roche, G. C. The bewildered society. *Imprimis* (Hillsdale College, Hillsdale, Michigan), January 1981, *10*, 1.

Stein, J., Ed. *The Random House Dictionary*. New York: Ballantine Books, 1978.

[6]

Professional Change and Marketing

Marketing: A Strategy for Power in Arenas of Competition

Christiana Gomboschi Wasserman

INTRODUCTION

The cost of health care in 1980 was $247 billion, up from a mere $27 billion in 1960. These costs are translated into approximately 10 percent of the Gross National Product, or $1,067 for each United States citizen (NLN, 1982). Some theoreticians and policy makers have identified "competition" as the panacea for these skyrocketing costs. Competition is defined as the struggle over scarce resources. The competitor, therefore, who offers the best product at the least price controls the consumer and the marketplace.

Success in the arena of competition depends on the ability to influence others into accepting one's own perspective and policies. In this arena, where questions of influence determine final outcomes, nursing's inputs and policies are often not solicited; or, if solicited, frequently they are ignored. An oft-touted slogan is, "Nursing's potential power is becoming nursing's death knell." Unless the profession embraces new and more effective strategies, nursing as an autonomous discipline will flounder. It will be dictated to by regulatory agencies, other health professions, other collective bargaining organizations, and uninformed consumer groups.

Marketing, a strategy long ignored by nurses and nursing, is a successful method for gaining the competitive edge. The concepts of marketing, applied in a planned and consistent manner, will result in the ability to influence others which yields *power*. It is a strategy which will assist in the implementation of nursing's policies and the attainment of nursing's goals.

ISSUES OF COMPETITION

The broad issues of competition facing the health care industry in general, and nursing specifically, are based on questions of access to the care-provider, fee-for-service versus prepaid health care, criteria for reimbursement, and illness versus wellness care and subsidization. Also critical are issues grounded in societal changes in values and expectations. These latter problems significantly affect professional expectations, values, and priorities in the health care delivery system.

Changes in beliefs about, and trends in, education, lifestyle, and societal imperatives have forced nursing to compete, albeit reluctantly, in the marketplace of education, employment, and legislation. The competition is fierce. It is more than optimistic to expect that nursing's current strategies will advance nursing goals.

What are the specific competition problems in nursing? Testifying before the Congressional Committee on Health and Long-Term Care, Davis (1981) presented an all-too-familiar litany. Nursing is among the ten lowest paid professions. A nurse makes an average salary of approximately $260 per week, or $13,500 annually. Compare this to a bus driver in the same city who makes $385 per week, or $20,000 annually. With this salary structure, can nursing really expect that women will either seek or stay in nursing as a career? The Department of Labor statistics identify that one out of every seven families is supported by a woman (Davis, 1981).

It is unrealistic to expect that the flight of women from nursing will be stemmed by the influx of men. Less than 5 percent of men are choosing nursing as a career (Davis, 1981). Men have traditionally sought careers promising prestige, advancement, and appropriate remuneration. Women are beginning to do the same. As a result, nursing is losing many of its best and brightest candidates to professional schools such as medicine, law, business, and engineering.

Some leaders in nursing seek advanced degrees which take them further from the bedside and patient care services. This creates elitism among nurses and is causing a schism between erstwhile ''colleagues'' at a time the profession can least afford such divisiveness.

The nurse who is seeking to expand the practice role is encountering real competition problems. The nurse-practitioner, not a particularly new role, is consistently encountering acceptance problems. *The Longitudinal Study of Nurse Practitioners*, conducted by the Health Resources Administration, documents that nurse practitioners frequently cite nonacceptance by various health providers as barriers to practice (Sultz, 1980).

The National League for Nursing Policy Bulletin presents some extremely troubling information. None of the Congressional bills addressing competition among health care providers include reference to nursing and nursing care (NLN, 1982). This is unfortunate in light of the fact that the most economical mix of health care services includes, and would be a boon to, nurse practitioners (NLN, 1982). Although the Rural Health Clinics Act of 1977 specifies nursing care reimbursement without supervision of a physician, this reimbursement is not yet a widespread practice (NLN, 1982). Indeed, the battle for reimbursement of nursing care, whether in-hospital or in private practice, is being fought hard, and for the most part, unsuccessfully. Currently, most nurses must be affiliated with a physician, either in practice or in a prepaid health organization, in order to admit clients/patients to a tertiary care hospital center. Even the private duty nurse, whose fee is covered by many insurance companies, does not have her or his fee reimbursed without a physician's written order.

What is the barrier to reimbursement for nursing care? Fagin (1982) identifies the primary reason as competition for physician dollars. As a result of this perceived competition, our colleagues in medicine have engaged in heavy and consistent lobbying against American Nurses' Association policies which might expand the access of nurses to clients in a one-to-one relationship. In addition, many of the areas in which nurses provide effective services are not reimbursable, or reimbursable only with physician approval: health promotion and disease prevention activities, nursing service in hospital centers as discrete activities, home health care, and health teaching.

The post-World War II baby boom generation is now past seeking their first college degree. The number of high school graduates is dropping significantly. The pool of potential eighteen-year-olds seeking admission to collegiate nursing programs has concomitantly diminished. Nursing should compete for the older adult student who is often seeking a post-high school degree for the first time. Nursing should identify areas where consumer demand is generating new health programs.

For example, a major New York state college recently announced the graduation of 16 Master's-prepared "patient advocates." Nurses view themselves as patient/client advocates, but nursing will lose that competition if others are not aware of this important role. Degrees in health education are proliferating. Where is nursing and its role in all this? Job counselors are advising high school guidance counselors, who face significant personnel cutbacks due to shrinking enrollments, to retool in order to change jobs and begin counseling outpatients and inpatients. What is nursing's role in this competition?

MARKETING CONCEPTS

Marketing may be defined as communicating with an audience or population in order to affect changes in opinions or behaviors. It is also designing a product or service so that it is easy to utilize, and distributing that service so that it is easy to find (Rados, 1981). The process of marketing, be it a service, product, or policy, results in command or control of scarce resources through voluntary exchange (Rados, 1981).

The implementation of a marketing plan requires the definition of four elements of marketing: the purpose, the objectives, the strategies, and the tactics. The results are disastrous if attempts at persuasion or promotion of a service or policy are made without clear identification of these elements first.

1. *Purpose:* The presenters of the service or policy must identify a clearly articulated and understood reason for the existence of the product, policy, or service. What does the organization want to accomplish by marketing this service or policy?

2. *Objectives:* What are the specific goals to be accomplished if the overall purpose is to be achieved? Are the goals critical to actualizing the philosophy, self-esteem, or purposes of the organization?

3. *Strategies:* What is the path to be followed to attain the purposes? What direction will the communication about the service or policy take? Will the marketer seek to call attention to the service or policy, to persuade the audience of the benefits of the service or policy, or to educate the audience about the service or policy?

4. *Tactics:* What programs are to be pursued to achieve the strategies? Will the marketer utilize one-to-one communication techniques, one-to-large population techniques, telecommunications, or print media?

The above four elements of marketing can further be subdivided. Kotler and Levy (1978) identify seven components of an effective marketing plan:

1. Product Definition: This is a broad definition of the service, policy, or product which emphasizes the basic consumer need(s) being served.

2. Definition of the Target Group: Because a policy, product, or service cannot be all things to all people, the marketer must identify the population which will be the primary or sole recipient of the communication.

3. Differentiated Marketing: In order to appeal to the target audience, different groups within that population may need to be communicated with in a different manner. The communications message must be reformulated so as to appeal to the differing factions within a target population.

4. Customer Behavior Analysis: This is a consideration and identification of the motives underlying the behavior of the target population.

5. Multiple Marketing Tools: What are the tools with which the organization will communicate its message to the target audience? Some avenues available are newsletters, news releases, campaign drives, annual reports, advertisements, educational events, public relations campaigns, and radio and television programs.

6. Integrated Market Planning: This is the overall coordination of policy and service as related to the specific item being marketed: the total responsibility for a specific item being marketed. The total reponsibility for a marketing campaign, however, should always rest solely with one individual.

7. Continuous Feedback and Periodic Audit: This is the ongoing process of assessing the environment, the competition, and the effectiveness of the marketing strategies in meeting the stated purpose.

Application of Marketing Strategy to Nursing Problem

Let's apply the marketing strategy identified above to a specific nursing problem, the image of nursing.

The purpose of the marketing plan is to improve or alter the current image of nursing. The objectives of the plan are (1) greater utilization of independent nurse practitioners as a result of the new image; (2) more independent and autonomous practice for nurses in acute care settings; (3) third-party reimbursement for discrete nursing activities regardless of where they are performed; or (4) altering existing practice acts to reflect current nursing roles. The strategies of the plan will focus on all three communication goals; will call attention to the skewed and inaccurate current image; will educate the target audience about the role and function of today's professional nurse; will persuade the target audience to seek the care and interventions which are uniquely nursing. The tactics utilized will focus on one-to-one communications with interdisciplinary health professionals; utilize print media, intra- and interprofessional as well as the popular journals; utilize limited use of television and radio broadcasts.

The product—nursing—will be difficult to define. What is needed is a definition which encompasses nursing's multifaceted specialties while presenting a role which the consumer can understand. Will the consumer be able to relate to (1) educational differentiations which have caused such intraprofessional turmoil; (2) issues of professional practitioners who are accountable only to clients and peers; or (3) portrayals of nurses as concerned caregivers who are with the client in times of emotional and physical stress and who care for the "whole" person? The definition of nursing will be marketed differently depending on the target population. A strategist would not present nursing's role and function and view of self as a profession to a physician in the same manner as to a nursing administrator. The definition and presentation would change if the target audience were allied health professionals, legislators, or consumers.

The tools with which to communicate about the role of nursing are diverse and plentiful. Public relations campaigns can widely present the role of nursing practitioners to both the consumer and interdisciplinary health professionals. In-house newsletters can address the expanded functions and roles of professional nurses. Public service announcements on radio and television can alert the public to new health care services being offered by a specific group of nurses in an area, or to educate the public about pending legislation and its impact not only on nursing but also on the consumer of patient care services. Press releases, especially in local papers, about nursing associations' policies and positions on issues related to health care are very effective in portraying the nurse as a formulator of quality care procedures and plans.

Assessing the motives of the target population is a much more difficult thing to do. How will consumers seek specific nursing professionals if they are not aware of their existence, or if they are not comfortable with the quality of care they perceive will be rendered? Do physicians hesitate about working with nurse practitioners because they are insecure in their own role, or because they are unfamiliar with the nurse practitioner's role, and/or because they resent the competition for control of the client and the subsequent financial reimbursement? Which organization will be responsible for the overall coordination of this plan to change nursing's image? Who within that organization will be ultimately responsible? Will the plan be directed by the national organization or by specialty groups, or by the nurses associations within each state?

It is critical to identify the parameters which will be used to evaluate the feedback about the strengths and weaknesses of the marketing campaign. Whose responses will be evaluated: consumers, nurses, allied health personnel? In what form will the evaluation mechanism be reviewed? Will reformulation of the marketing strategy depend only on letters and telephone calls, or on survey responses from practitioners, or will the evaluation be assessed based on the number of bills successfully "gotten through" the local legislature?

SUMMARY

Society's resources, be they technologies, dollars, or people, are becoming more and more scarce. In the face of these diminishing resources, the protagonist with a logical, well thought out marketing strategy will win the competition. Other disciplines have long recognized this fact, and acted accordingly. Only now is nursing coming to realize that without a comparable, if not better marketing strategy, the profession will have no voice in the precincts of power and policy. We hope it is not too late for nursing. We hope the profession will be able to articulate a clear and cohesive strategy for its goals with the implementation of a marketing plan.

REFERENCES

Davis, C. Nursing shortage and its impact on care for the elderly. Hearing before the Subcommittee on Health and Long-term Care of the Select Committee on Aging. 96th Congress, 2nd Session. August 20, 1980. Com. Pub. #96–255. U.S. Government Printing Office, Washington, D.C., 1981.

Fagin, C. Nursing's pivotal role in achieving competition in health care. In *From accommodation to self-determination: Nursing's role in the development of health care policy.* Kansas: American Nurses' Association, 1982.

Kotler, P., & Levy, S. J. Broadening the concept of marketing. In P. J. Montana (Ed.), *Marketing in nonprofit organizations.* New York: AMACOM, 1978.

National League for Nursing. Competition in health care. *NLN Policy Bulletin,* January 18, 1982.

Rados, D. L. *Marketing for non-profit organizations.* Boston: Auburn House Publishing Co., 1981.

Sultz, H. A., Zielezny, M., & Smith, N. *Longitudinal study of nurse practitioners, Phase III.* DHEW Publication No. HRA 80–2. U.S. Department of Health, Education, and Welfare, Public Health Service, Health Resources Administration, Bureau of Health Manpower, Division of Nursing, U.S. Government Printing Office, Washington, 1980.

SUGGESTED READINGS

Fox, K. F. A., & Kotler, P. The marketing of social causes: The first 10 years. *Journal of Marketing*, 1980, *44*, 24–33.

Frorbe, D. J. The marketing process. In A. Marriner (Ed.), *Contemporary nursing management*. St. Louis: C. V. Mosby, 1982.

Romera, R., & Levitt, R. Packaging the package. *American Journal of Nursing*, 1981, *81*(1), 106.

Sawyer, G. Elements of a strategy. *Managerial Planning*, 1981, *29*(6), 3–5, 9.

Starr, P. Changing the balance of power in American medicine. *Milbank Memorial Fund Quarterly/Health and Society*, 1980, *58*(1), 166–172.

Quelch, J. A. Marketing principles and the future of preventive health care. *Milbank Memorial Fund Quarterly/Health and Society*, 1980, *58*(2), 310–347.

Nursing: Societal Discontent and Professional Change*

Myrtle K. Aydelotte

INTRODUCTION

Wherever there are human beings, nursing will be practiced. Nursing will be needed "to put the constitution in such a state that it will have no disease or that it can recover from disease" (Nightingale, 1894, p. 1). Birthing, living, and dying are experiences of human life, and as long as there is human life there will be the need to care for individuals undergoing those experiences. This is the truth about nursing and its survival.

*This paper was given at the Fourth Annual Elizabeth S. Soule Lecture at the University of Washington, School of Nursing, Washington, D.C. on October 7, 1982.

The problem is not the survival of nursing. The problem lies in so-cietal discontent and in needed changes in nursing practice. Nursing is an occupation undergoing professionalization and responding at the same time to changes in its external environment. Many of those changes appear to threaten advances in professionalization of the occupation. But as those forces are studied, opportunity presents itself to bring about changes which will benefit nurses and the public.

THE REALITIES: CHANGES IN SOCIETY

Various attitudes are observed among the citizenry today. Readily observable is the cynicism expressed by various individuals and groups of society toward the private sector and the social attitude of government. Although the general public continues to express no loss of confidence in the free enterprise system upon which our society has been structured, many continue to see the need for some form of regulation to control business abuses. It is the amount of regulation and its placement that continue to be debatable. Many believe that at the federal level there is too much regulation and insufficient confidence and reliance placed on local government. A large number of citizens see the federal government as pinched and overextended; yet, when proposals are made for rebalance or redistribution of money, programs, and power, the cynical lack of confidence in government to do this becomes apparent. The public hostility toward the tax structure and expressed need to make it more equitable, less complex, and more understandable are readily apparent. There appears to be growing antagonism among government, business, and labor groups.

Basic to this attitude of cynicism and lack of confidence in government's ability to address concerns and redress them is a very fundamental human deficit in our society. Our capacity to reach consensus on major policy questions has deteriorated. Present in society today are well-organized and uncompromising single-issue forces made up of special interest groups. These groups are using political techniques to make their resentment and opposition felt. There is an unwillingness to accommodate to the common good and to sacrifice for the larger interest. The tenacious holding on to self-interest and self-serving goals creates a situation that paralyzes the machinery by which policy is formed. Sometimes it is difficult to develop policy reasonably acceptable to divergent interests and still in keeping with the common good.

Closely associated with these special interest groups, but different, are those sectors in our society who are seeking a return to "traditionalism." Although these sectors are highly organized, there are fluctuations even within in the movement toward traditionalism as well as differences of opinion about what to emphasize in traditionalism. The development of the traditionalism trend may have various roots—shifts in religious emphasis, increased diversity of religions, and the failure of our social institutions to keep pace with technological, economical, and social changes. The social institutions of the family, schools, churches, and businesses have been greatly altered. Many have not made accommodations or alterations to societal changes. The lack of business to accommodate to new styles of life, to family changes, and to workforce changes is one example.

This leads to the observation that these societal changes are turning us into a nation characterized by great diversity of values, beliefs, traditions, and rituals. These changes are involving us in a whirlwind of debate and argument. How our energy can be harnessed so that we can agree about the "common good" and find means to accomplish it is today's challenge.

One of the most striking observations in society today is the change in the labor force. Dramatic shifts are occurring. The percentage of professionals is increasing while the percentage of blue-collar and farm workers is decreasing. The proportion of highly skilled workers is greater in relation to low-skilled workers. Within the next 15 years, there will be a decline in young persons, age 18 to 21 years. This reduction in young workers is taking place when the need for college-trained personnel is high and on the rise, so much so that a labor shortage may occur in the 1980s.

The workforce is becoming older and better educated. The average age of the population in 1982 is 30 years; by the year 2000 it will be 35 years. The population aged 25 to 44 years will be the most rapidly growing segment for the next 12 years.

The workforce is also including more women, more Spanish-speaking people, and more blacks. It has been predicted that within the next 10 years, 61 percent of women of working age will be in the workforce.

Major changes are occurring in the type of work to be done as a result of changes in technology and information systems and the shift in manufacturing to nonagricultural nonmanufacturing. There are other marked rearrangements in the employment scene. Decentralization of industry is taking place, and new types of industry are developing.

The worker of today and tomorrow is more likely to live in rural areas, elect later retirement, demand flexible working hours, ask for job sharing or part-time instead of layoffs, and less likely to be a member of a labor union. An employee is likely to be in competition with an older employee rather than a younger one, since we are moving into a three- and four-generation workforce. These are the results of complex fundamental forces in the demography of the labor resources which cannot be halted.

Closely related to the change in labor force is the trend in economic growth. Though shaky and subject to rapid fluctuations, the current prediction is positive, but slow, economic growth. The expectation is that less funds will be provided by the federal government in the immediate future for meeting the social problems of the nation. An increased proportion of funds will be needed for energy. Stimulation of the economy is being encouraged through mechanisms of competition and limited regulation. The economy for the near future is described as "characterized by slow growth, disinflation, high unemployment, fluctuating prices, and continued high interest rates (*Environmental Assessment*, 1983, p. 3).

THE REALITIES: THE WORK ENVIRONMENT FOR NURSES

As one examines the social, political, and economical forces within society at large, one begins to question what impact this does have upon nurses and their opportunities to practice. What are the forces of changes and predicted changes in the health field? Nurses today compose a large workforce. In what form and mode will they survive?

The majority of nurses are employed in hospitals. In this author's opinion—and this will be referred to later—they should be viewed and should view themselves as *salaried professionals*. Since the employment of nurses is primarily in the hospital sector, the author suggests that the profession examine what is predicted, or suggested, for hospitals to use as alternative management and governance strategies. The strategies for change are numerous. Results that can be expected are these:

- Health care institutions will become increasingly diversified and the range of services provided will become more comprehensive and broader in scope.
- Health care corporations will continue to develop and will include several types of institutions under one major corporate structure, but growth will soon level off.
- Long-range planning, flexibility, responsiveness to environmental change, and accountability of the various professionals and boards of trustees will become increasingly important.
- Competition for funding and for patients and clients between institutions, individual professionals, and organized professional groups will increase. There will be an increase in the diversity of types of organizations providing services.

- Underwriters of health benefit plans and employers will demand improved services, efficiency, and economy in return for payment of health benefits—the promotion and use of innovative services will be sought.
- Technology and scientific innovation will continue, but they will be directed toward specific groups and effectiveness will be emphasized.
- In response to consumer demand, health services will evaluate services in order to eliminate redundancy, minimize cost, promote quality, and emphasize cost-effectiveness.
- Emphasis will be placed on health promotion, maintenance of individual worker performance, and quality of life in the community.
- Control of health care spending, that is, the limitation of financial resources, will be the driving force to make changes in the field.
- The management of human resources will change. Concern will be directed toward wise utilization, effectiveness, economy, and efficiency. Each professional and service occupation will redefine and clarify its roles. Fewer different professions and workers will result with great differentiation within each group. Competition for funds and clients and patients within and between professionals will intensify. The number of employed professionals will increase.

If nurses examine these statements for their implications for the profession, nursing can see that great opportunities—as well as challenges and threats—for nurses are present.

First of all, by 1990, the number of physicians will be increased to such an extent that a surplus of 70,000 is predicted. The Harris Hall Poll of 1,814 physicians conducted for the Kaiser Family Foundation stated that physicians reported that they are having trouble practicing where they want to be, that many are changing hours and services, and the weekly visits for new patients are down for the first quarter of 1982 ("U.S. Health Care Costs," 1982). If physicians are experiencing this difficulty now, the problem will become even more acute by 1990. One can speculate that physicians will increase competition among themselves and with all other health workers.

Second, one can predict that the role of the chief hospital executive or corporate hospital executive will become increasingly powerful. The hospital executive probably will manage a wider range of institutions and be granted a greater degree of authority by the board of trustees. Within the hospital as well as other types of organizations, the relations between the professionals and specific bureaucratic individuals will become increasingly important. The power of the bureaucratic structure will continue to determine the strategy making among and within the professions. The drive for professionalization of the aspiring health occupations will become more pronounced, and the introduction of technology, especially that dealing with information, will demand new skills of professionals.

Third, the tasks of leadership in all fields will become more difficult. Leaders will require greater breadth, knowledge, and sophistication. No longer will decisions be made without reference to framework, analysis, and a systematic approach to the gathering of data and information. Decisions will have far-reaching effects on many individuals, not a small core of people. Therefore, the decisions made by leadership groups in the professions and bureaucracies will impact greatly on many because of the rippling effect.

Fourth, the driving force behind all changes in the delivery and health and medical services will be the limitation of financial resources. The amount of money spent on health care will increase very little. Growth of funds will be slow, and consequently, the containment of costs will become even more imperative. New ways to economize will be sought, including the examination of the effectiveness of personnel and the possible elimination of some workers in the field. For this reason, the opportunity for the growth of labor unions in the health care sector is even greater than that now present.

Fifth, nurses will have many different types of settings in which to practice. In spite of this change, however, the major employers will continue to be hospitals and hospital corporations. As nurses develop more experience and sophistication in both nursing and management, a number will engage in their own group practices and business.

Sixth, professions will move into tasks of role clarification, differentiation, and structuring of the occupations, employing the techniques of competition and negotiation. Each health profession will seek new markets. The competition among professionals will be great—competition for talented individuals to enter the profession, for educational funds, for markets, and for societal sanction. This competition will be partly balanced by recognition that cooperation with other groups is essential for survival.

NURSES AND THE NURSING PROFESSION: HOPES AND FEARS

The author has briefly examined the social, economic, and political forces impinging on the health field. It is now appropriate to look at how nurses and the nursing profession will fare in the environment created by those forces. The author believes nursing will survive. The question is: in what form will the occupation survive? Will it move into full maturity or will it be constrained in its development? Will the professionalization process under which it has been going be impeded or will the process accelerate?

Professionalization

Professionalization is the process by which an occupation moves toward a special form of control called a profession. In our society, a profession is a social class which has the approval and sanction of society as a whole. Professions arise as unique products of the division of labor. They are open to individuals from all social and economic classes in our society in that those who gain entrance to the professions are from those classes. Our society has accepted movement into professions as a form of acceptable social mobility and social differentiation.

Although the transition of an occupation to a profession is not a uniform process, there are certain elements in the process that are recognizable. There is a development of group consciousness and the development of a successful ideology to which the group adheres. A privileged position is secured for the group by the political and economic elite of the group through their use of persuasion, negotiation, coalition building, justification of the legitimacy for the professional control, and the construction of ties with the powerful or rising classes. A special body of dominant experts in the occupation constructs the parameters and characteristics of the prevailing ideology.

Barber states that there are four attributes which characterize a profession:

1. A high degree of generalized and systematic knowledge.
2. A primary orientation to the community interest rather than self-interest.
3. A high degree of self-control of behavior, achieved through an ideology and internalization of code of ethics.
4. A set of rewards which are monetary and honorary in nature. Honors are highly valued. (Johnson, 1972)

In the transition of an occupation to a profession, special and exclusive knowledge held by its members is essential. It is powerful in establishing control by the professionals and in the development of the markets of the professionals. The knowledge possesses a cognitive rationality and yet contains an esoteric quality. Since not everyone can use the knowledge, for they do not have it (it is not common knowledge), those who do possess the knowledge have control of their professional activities. This negotiation of *cognitive exclusiveness* results in the creation of social and economic dependence on the profession. The emergence of special occupational skills, dependent on the knowledge exclusive to the practitioner, leads to the creation of a dependent market. The tacit understanding of their exclusiveness by the practitioners creates a social distance between the practitioners and others. The practitioners become a social class unto themselves.

Currently, the nursing occupation, though moving toward professionalization, is experiencing difficulties in the transition. Many of these difficulties are known. There is a limited body of tested knowledge underlying the practice. Not enough basic clinical nursing research has been conducted, and what has been done is not applied with sufficient frequency to make an impact. Credibility gaps between the ideal prescriptive theory taught by faculty in educational programs and the objective reality of the knowledge used by those in the practice world exists. The work groups in nursing are segmented and hold varying values and concerns. Practitioners and theorists are not in accord on what is significant in practice, and unfortunately, collaboration and support for each other are sometimes lacking between those two important groups. Fine-tuned prescriptive theory and experimental learning of clinical experts in the practice field are ignored at times. Yet these are the very ones who provide the framework for practice. The logic of the field, referred to as the nursing process, has become procedural rather than characterized by intellectual inquiry (Henderson, 1982). But the most serious problem is the general recognition of a distinctive, exclusive commodity, the *professional nurse.*

Perhaps the author seems critical of nursing, but it is an attempt to be honest. Given the environment of today, nursing will continue to be perceived as semiprofessional and technical unless certain changes are made. In order to become professional, the nursing occupation requires an educational base acquired in a university or college and representing a minimum of a baccalaureate degree. The knowledge base and the ideology provided those who enter the field must be such that the superiority of the graduate is firmly established and unquestioned by all, thereby eliminating any other competing product.

The recruitment, selection, and training of entrants into the profession cannot be overemphasized.

But also we must look forward to the proper utilization of the graduates, the delineation of new roles, and the differentiation of occupation into support groups to the professional, their accountability, and their training. The individual who is trained as a professional must be perceived as such and treated as such.

STRATEGIES FOR MATURATION OF THE PROFESSION

It is essential to recognize that the control of the occupation, that is, the development of the profession, is gained by two major means: access to the field and the creation of a special market for professional services. In regard to access to the field, the universities are gatekeepers to the professions. It is the faculty of a professional school that determines who enters that profession. In nursing, the public is confused by the setting forth of varying and uneven "products" from three types of schools. There is a failure to demarcate the graduate who is a professional from the others. Academic leaders, nursing managers, and practitioners must join together to identify the general and specialized knowledge that is needed for professional practice. Not only should this knowledge include the broad spectrum of health, health promotion, counseling, illness care, and the knowledge required for specialized services in nursing, but it should stress general principles and their applications and be so difficult that it is outside the grasp of anyone with less than a college degree. Although the main object is to develop an educational excellence in problem-solving ability and competence so that others with less academic preparation are viewed as technicians, the secondary object is to designate knowledge base and skills required by individuals in need of professional nursing services. The services which result should benefit the public. These services should be oriented to the complexity of nursing care required during illness or to situations which may lead to illness. It is necessary for us to identify the difference between professional nursing services and personal care.

Efforts must also be made to bond the students to the members in the professional community and to the ideology they espouse through an intense socialization process. Included in the ideology are references and beliefs concerned with ethical principles, community, self-governance, and careers. The bonding is fostered through affective relationships in the mentoring process and through the use of language. The object is to bring about identification with the collective, to ensure support and loyalty to each other, to the nursing field, and to the clientele to be served. Sufficient homogeneity in the ideology is desired to move us forward as a collective. Nurses use negotiations and persuasion in seeking to make legitimate the advances toward cognitive exclusiveness.

The strategy that the author proposes for resolving access to the profession is one for the leadership of the occupation. The nurse leadership in universities, in influential centers where fine nursing management exists, and among selected nurse practitioners (staff nurses and clinical specialists) must come together to address and resolve this question. Patients, clients, employers, and the general public will continue to be confused about who is a professional nurse, what services that individual can provide, and what sanctions and rewards are in order, unless the nursing leadership rationally solves this problem of designing and preparing the professional product and the support groups in nursing. Nursing leadership in all schools must first agree on how the occupation will be structured. The strategies to be used by these leaders must be negotiation, persuasion, rationalization for the common good, trade-offs, and mechanisms for saving face for the current varied practitioners in the field. The object is to design what is needed in the occupation and the plan of how to get there. Some of the social, economic, and political influences currently operating in our society will facilitate action; others will impede action. The major influence which is detering us is our inability to come to consensus for the common good for both the public and nurses.

The second set of strategies deal with the creation of a market for nursing services. In nursing, both the producer (the nurse) and the employer (the hospital or agency) define needs for services and how these are met. The nurse with the patient and client defines nursing needs, while the employer is the consumer of the expert services of the nurse only indirectly. The relationship of consumption of services indirectly by employers is true of most salaried professionals.

Professional autonomy for the salaried professional may be impaired, but it is not eliminated. Autonomy resides within the technical and scientific knowledge of the professionals and the exclusiveness of their services. The problem for nursing resides in the perception of the staff nurse as an employee in the sense of the working classes, rather than a salaried professional who directs her or his own work, makes clinical decisions, and manages the content, pace, and selection of services to be granted clients and patients. The past practices used in the study of nursing which emphasized task definition, task arrangements, simplicity, and efficiency have contributed to the perception of nursing practice as routinized, low-level, and nonintellectual work.

Some nursing activities have also created questions on the part of employers about loyalty to the institution. The structure of nursing departments has been patterned after the models of industrial production rather than after models of professional departments existing in corporations, educational institutions, and scientific institutes. Restructuring of nursing departments is needed in order to provide the kind of environment in which staff nurses can operate as professionals and be treated as such. Staff nurses who operate in settings where they receive the support, rewards, and opportunities of professionals become professionals, in a self-fulfilling prophecy.

Many people in occupations that aspire to professionalism are salaried employees, and their employers are well-organized. Since many of the aspiring professionals believe or perceive that their autonomy is reduced by the action of their employers, they place great emphasis upon contracts for services. The professional organization operates more as a labor union than as a professional body, and is seen as a union by employers. This perception of the nature of the professional organization creates additional strains in the relationship between employers and salaried professionals contributing to the impediment of the professionalization process.

Further, the professional who becomes an administrator in a bureaucracy experiences not only role conflict, but also professional identity problems. Unless the structure is kept flat, and the individual's management techniques, strategy, and rituals reflect professional understanding, support, and concerns, the administrator will confront credibility problems with the professionals in the field in which he or she is trained.

What can the salaried professional do to develop the market for his or her services? A market is created through the development of superior services—these services must be distinctive, and must be offered by an individual who is well-trained and socialized into the professional community. Superiority of services eliminates the use of competing individuals or products. In nursing, this will result in the elimination of substituting less well-trained persons for professional nurses, and the elimination of "pulling" nurses off one nursing specialty to provide service to patients on another. It can lead to the creation of competition between consumers (that is, employers) of nursing.

The superiority of services is created not only by the performance of graduates and their impact on an institution but also through the use of ideological persuasion with influential groups and elite members of the community. Leading practitioners holding credentials and honors, as well as academicians, researchers, and nurse managers must plan strategies by which they align themselves in different ways with powerful persons in the community. The author urges nurses to become involved in community affairs, seeking a role on committees, in political parties, on various boards, and on study groups. In all of these, the presentation of the individual on these bodies *as a nurse* is essential to further the image of the nurse as professional.

Nurses must look at ways of identifying the production of income, either in agencies or institutions or through group practice, with the expectation that there be a fair return of earnings to the nurse as a producer. Too often, nursing departments and units have been viewed as cost centers, when in essence, they are income-generating centers as well. The value of the income produced by keeping the census of a hospital high and the activities of a clinic heavy cannot be overestimated. The value of a hospital bed is reflected in the quarrels of medical staff as to which service the bed will be assigned as well as the concern expressed when nursing staff is not available to open a new nursing unit. Nursing is not credited with being income-producing. The author suggests that nursing work on the problem of identifying the monetary value of the service and push for its recognition.

Nurses also need to look for new markets for their services. The author is convinced that there are many persons who would purchase nursing services if they are privately organized and controlled by nurses and if nurses had but the courage and the willingness to run the financial risk of such an operation. Nurses are competent to run supplemental agencies, at-home gerontological services, counseling clinics, obesity clinics, and the like. Nurses need to become entrepreneurs and set up their own businesses.

The third set of strategies nursing should put in place are those that deal with educational policies. Nurses need to continue the practice of social mobility by allowing persons in our society to advance, through education, according to their own merit and talents. The wealth of a nation and the conditions of its people depend upon the skill, dexterity, and knowledge of its people. The supply of a highly educated people, from all sectors of a nation, is an absolute requirement. There needs to be federal and state support for the education of individuals who enter occupations that are socially important but who receive upon graduation a low level of compensation. In planning their strategy, nurses should align themselves with these groups and assist in the presentation of the case for funds to support individuals seeking careers in these fields and the institutions where the education is provided.

The fourth set of strategies are structured around policies needed by the labor force. Although the percentage of women in the workforce has steadily increased over the last 50 years, women are still treated as outsiders. Many political leaders express the opinion that women are the major contributors to the vast employment problem, but those politicians fail to acknowledge the change in the structure of the household, the impact of technology on household work and management, and the changes in standards of living which require two-income families. Neither is there general recognition in our society that women's work has equal value to men's. The issues relate to equity, child care, maternity leave, and working conditions. Nursing groups must address these issues along with others in order to create policies which are progressive and by which both men and women benefit. The improvement in the quality of the "working" life of all persons needs improvement. Special attention is needed to adapt work patterns to changing societal attitudes regarding work and to an increase in self-direction, pacing, and scheduling. The inflexibility of work policies and the inequities in salaries and conditions for work for men and women are leading to frustration and nonproduction. The strategies to be employed are those of coalition building, political action, negotiation, litigation, and persuasion.

The fifth set of strategies is directed toward changes in the field regarding the nursing organizations. While the relationships between and among the nursing organizations have improved over the last few years, there are persistent strains founded in competition for power, socialization as women, diversity of interests, and isolation from the mainstream in the health field. Competition for the dues dollar from nurses will increase, and unless there is a change in thinking, payment of dues will be considered a luxury. The socialization of women, which has resulted in lack of team-building skills and hesitancy to recognize women as intelligent and valuable authorities, has contributed to difficulty in collaboration with each other on major issues in the nursing field. Nurses need to recognize that in every nursing organization there are hierarchies of influence that socialization of the entrants to the profession and socialization of nurses as women brings to bear upon actions and this anarchy. Chaska (1983) speaks eloquently on this point in *The Nursing Profession: A Time to Speak*, and Styles (1982) discusses it in her recent book, *On Nursing: Toward a New Endowment*, where she describes the qualities of professionhood. Personal ambitions should not compete with professional organizational goals. Can nurses not bring together the organizations in the profession and present, at least to the public and to other professions, a stand which represents unity of thought and respect? Nursing needs unity on educational preparation, credentialing, research, and utilization. Can nurses also urge growth, support, endorsement, and sponsorship of the young in the profession, rather than handicap them by asking them to "stand the test" and endure the trials that others in older generations experienced? The true value of leadership is reflected in the leaders that an individual has produced. Strategies for changes in organized nursing rest upon the skills, influence, and coalition building of those in positions within those organizations. To make changes requires patience, a sense of timing, persuasion, and influence, and a willingness to experience failure and then to try again. The environment of today, which contains attitudes in which consensus building is tough, makes achievement of this goal difficult. But the achievement is essential in the maturing of the nursing profession.

The employment of approaches to meet these five sets of strategies which are needed in order to survive—not as technical and semiprofessional, but as capable of full maturation as professionals—involve interaction with powerful groups in other professions, the government, and elite groups in the communities in which nurses live and work. It also charges nurses to examine how they can interact among themselves in supportive and productive ways.

Among the powerful professions and groups with whom nurses interact and with whom interactions should increase are physicians, hospital administrators, and trustees. These three sets of individuals exert not only influence in the work environment but in the community as well. Working with these individuals can be difficult. The difficulty arises from events that have occurred in the history of nursing, medicine, and hospital administration as well as in the education of individuals in these fields. The knowledge, language, culture, orientation, and authority of each differs. Physicians, trustees, and hospital administrators are often men; nurses are most often women.

Cooperation among all groups can lead to an improvement of services to patients and clients and to economy, efficiency, and effectiveness of the systems of delivery. A second object is the promotion of mutual professional interests and those in the field of health. As mature individuals, nurses can recognize that there are subjects on which nurses will differ, and about which nurses will attempt to persuade others to believe. In spite of differences, there are agenda items on which all health professionals can work.

The agenda items include changes in women's work; development of careers and expectations for women that are similar to men; the problems, demands, stresses, and strains on each profession; changes occurring in each field; language differences; impact of technology; the valuation of knowledge and experience of nurses; and many others.

Nurses have much to gain from working together in a fashion that conveys commitment to the services of patients and clients and to each other. Nurses need to develop a set of attitudes which are directed toward the following:

- Development of trust, respect, and openness
- Recognition of conflict and confrontation
- Learning of new languages, new symbols, and values
- Change in leadership style when needed
- Recognition of need for support and approval

In the development of this attitude set, nurses can share educational experiences and professional orientation. Nurses can also examine the nature of work in hospitals and health care institutions and its meaning for employees. Nurses can study how to reduce unhealthy competition and impersonalization in the work environment. The opportunity to challenge the organizational norms and habits that exist will arise, and nurses can establish new values and beliefs or recommit themselves to the old. The overriding purpose of nurses being there—caring for people—should become apparent to all.

Nurses can also apply what they know about organizational structure to create an opportunity for certain changes to take place. Organizational structures that introduce interactions and testing of perceptions need to be developed in hospitals and health care institutions. There are two types of changes: one relates to all institutional or interdepartmental rearrangements; the other concerns the nursing department.

The environmental forces that are buffeting the health care field are making this an opportune time for such dialogue. Nursing leadership should take the lead in establishing the interaction. It will be difficult at first, but nurses must keep in mind that the relations will not improve without discussion, together, of these concerns and an understanding of nursing and the value of its full maturation.

THE FUTURE AND A VISION

This chapter has reviewed political, economic, and social influences in society and the changes they are making in the health field. These changes challenge nurses to consider the strategies by which nursing will meet those changes and the kinds of interaction in which they should engage. Nurses must have within themselves an idea of what full maturation of nursing and the profession means. To the author it means the provision of an exclusive service greatly needed by our society, which rests on a distinct discipline, a code of ethics, a credentialing system, and a commitment to those served. This end is within nursing's reach, and nurses must reach for it. Without it, society will be poorer—less nursed, less cared for, and less cherished.

REFERENCES

Chaska, N. L. (Ed.) *The Nursing Profession: A Time to Speak.* New York: McGraw-Hill, 1983.
Environmental Assessment. Overview: 1983 Prototype. The Hospital Research and Educational Trust, 840 North Lake Shore Drive, Chicago, Illinois 60611.

Henderson, V. The nursing process—is the title right? *Journal of Advanced Nursing*, 1982, *7*, 103–109.
Johnson, T. J. *Professions and power*. London: MacMillan Press, Ltd., 1972.
Nightingale, F. *Notes on nursing: What it is, and what it is not*. New York: Appleton and Company, 1894.
Styles, M. M. *On Nursing: Toward a New Endowment*. St. Louis: C. V. Mosby, 1982.
U.S. health care costs increased 15% last year. *The Wall Street Journal*, July 27, 1982, p. 3.

SUGGESTED READINGS

Aiken, L., & Gortner, S. R. (Eds.) *Nursing in the 1980s: Crisis, opportunities, challenges*. Philadelphia: J. B. Lippincott Co., 1982.
American Medical Association. Report on the council on long-range planning and development. *The Environment of Organized Medicine*. American Medical Association, 1982.
Arygis, C., & Schon, D. A. *A theory in practice: Increasing professional effectiveness*. San Francisco: Jossey-Bass Publishers, 1974.
Bardi, C. A. Job sharing alternatives draw nurses back to the hospital. *Hospitals*, June 16, 1981, *55*, 12.
Begun, W. *Professionalism and the public interest: Price and quality in optometry*. Cambridge, Mass.: The MIT Press, 1981.
Bok, D. *The President's report*. Cambridge, Mass.: Harvard University, 1980–1981.
Freidson, E. *Professional dominance: The social structure of medical care*. Chicago: Aldine Publishing Co., 1970.
Gibson, R. M., & Waldo, D. R. National health expenditures, 1981. *Health Care Financing Review*, September 1982, *4*(I), 5–9.
Kessler-Harris, A. Working women: Myths and realities. *The New York Times*, August 18, 1982.
Larson, M. S. *The rise of professionalism: A sociological analysis*. Berkeley-Los Angeles-London: The University of California Press, 1977.
Lippman, T. W. America's workforce rapidly changing. *The Hartford Courant*, August 17, 1982, Section D, p. 1.
Mechanic, D., & Aiken, L. Sounding board: A cooperative agenda for medicine and nursing. *The New England Journal of Medicine*, 1982, *307*(12), 747–750.
Moore, W. E. *The professions: Roles and rules*. New York: Russell Sage Foundation, 1970.
Pines, B. Y. *The traditionalist movement that is sweeping grassroots America*. New York: William Morrow and Co., 1982.
Schiff, F. W. (Ed.) *Looking ahead: Identifying key economic issues for business and society in the 1980s*. Worcester, Mass.: The Hefferman Press, 1980.
Trend toward multiple hospital systems aimed at lower cost health care study. *Hospitals*, November 16, 1981, *55*, 45.

Vance, C. N. Women leaders: Modern day heroines or social deviants? *Image*, December 1979, 37–41.

Wald, M. L. The workplace in transition. *The New York Times*, September 5, 1982, Section 11, p. 1.

Games of Power and Politics: Trade Unions and Nurses' Rights

Elaine E. Beletz

INTRODUCTION

In the midst of record high unemployment, slow economic recovery, and numerous health care cutbacks, the operative shortage and increasing demand for professional nurses appears anomalous in an otherwise depressing economic milieu. Labor unions have been most affected by the current economy. At present, organized labor represents only 20 percent of the labor force and the proportion represented has been on the decline since the late 1970s. Numerous newspaper accounts address the loss of power and clout of the labor unions, the "give-backs" at the bargaining table, the massive layoffs, and the poor prospects for increasing union membership through organizing activities.

The American trade union movement has been referred to as "business unionism" and, as such, labor unions must increase their sagging membership to stay operative. Increasingly since 1974, professional nurses—because of their numbers and relatively low degree of organization for collective bargaining purposes—have been targeted as the panacea for maintaining the viability of trade unions.

A recent decision by the National Labor Relations Board (NLRB) may be of some benefit to trade union organizations. In August 1982, the NLRB reversed its policy and indicated that they will no longer investigate the truth or falsity of statements made by parties in an organizing campaign. Previous to this decision, election results would be set aside as an unfair labor practice if campaign literature contained numerous misrepresentations of facts. Generally, the aim of the election atmosphere was to provide a nearly ideal arena equivalent to those of "laboratory conditions" (General Shoe Co., 1948). This would allow the employee to have uninhibited freedom of choice which would be rational and based on the arguments presented (Getman et al., 1975).

The labor union organizer from start to finish concentrates on appeals to emotion. The drive to unionize is imbued with an emotional fervor designed to capture the loyalties of the group and individual and to create solidarity with union purpose.

In light of the recent NLRB decision and labor's desire to organize nurses, it is the intent of this author to address important issues and questions which nurses would consider in the event of a trade union organization drive.

THE TRADE UNION

To the average employee, a trade union is perceived as a powerful or possibly destructive organization (depending on viewpoint) made up of a group of people, who negotiate wages and hours, handle grievances, and lead strikes. In reality, however, a trade union is a political machine; it is politically operated by a political leadership created on a foundation of patronage available at the national level. It is a conflict organization with its own ideology, traditions, and loyalties, and its leadership focuses on maintaining and improving the image and power of the union (Lester, 1958). Socialism was an important force in developing union ideology and vestiges of its influence remain (Rees, 1977).

TRADE UNION MEMBERSHIP

The American labor movement has always been predominantly representative of manual workers. As recently described,

> AFL-CIO's basic commitment remains to the white male worker in a collective bargaining unit. In a few unions, women and blacks have been appointed to symbolic positions where they exercise little, if any, internal influence. (Hill, 1982)

Though many of the local unions may be headed by blacks or women, only one of the 101 national unions affiliated with the AFL-CIO is headed by a black and none by a woman. Of the approximately 15 million members, blacks constitute 23 percent, women 29 percent; and of the 35-member governing executive committee, there is one black and two women, one of whom is black (Hill, 1982). It would certainly not appear that the needs of women have been a focal point of the labor movement.

THE ORGANIZING DRIVE

During an organizing drive, rational and logical facts tend to be downplayed in favor of appeals to emotion. Yet an understanding of the labor union's ideology, commitment to professionals, women, and minorities is crucial for an informed decision. These factors will inevitably come to the forefront in developing union demands, determining outcomes, and forwarding a stance on issues.

Concepts of social justice, redistribution of income, and eradication of elitist barriers are intrinsic to union ideology. The record of poor performance for promoting social justice and impact on the nation's wealth has been well documented.

The elitist barrier concept separates society into different groups. Examples of such barriers may be educational credentials, licenses, and salaries. In contrast to a manual laborer, or nonprofessional worker, the nurse is designated as a professional; this status has been achieved through a long period of education which leads to a license to practice. The nurse can be classified as elitist in that he or she has different qualifications than the average worker in the previously mentioned groups. Some members of society and the profession recognize that what nurses do is unique and no other group can do it. Yet this purview is not held by all; for instance, take note of the substitution for professional nursing by practical nurses and aides.

The professional nurse license may be perceived as an obstacle by substitute workers for nurses. This perception is particularly important for trade unions who represent large numbers of unlicensed health care workers. The registered nurse license may be deemed an impediment toward advancing both the job interests and economic rewards for their nonlicensed members. Control of the registered nurse is pivotal for these unions since he or she is key to the salary structure for most hospital employees. Additionally, control of the professional nurse may allow for expansion of the roles of nonprofessional nursing personnel and thereby allow for the reduction of wage differences between the two categories of employees. Of course, if you expand the role of the substitute worker, you have less need to hire the professional.

At the American Federation of Teachers convention (AFT) in July

1982, a resolution was submitted and adopted entitled, "Individual Licenses for Registered Professional Nurses." This resolution called upon the nurses and health professionals local to continue to support individual licensure for registered nurses and disapprove the substitution of institutional licensure which purports to do away with individual licensure. This action raises several questions. Why was only the local union to be supportive of individual licensure? Why not the national union since they are part of it? Have there been any other public positions taken by any other local or national unions or the AFL-CIO itself? If they have not taken positions, will each of these levels take public positions now, or is it politically judicious to remand it to an embryonic local union?

As professional nurses know, value systems and philosophies are keys to behavior. Representation by trade unions—even if they call themselves professional—connotes a commitment to the labor movement and its fundamental tenets and ideology and therefore characterizes one as a trade unionist. Collective bargaining is only one tool of representation, and should not be confused or equated with—or provide support for—the trade union movement as a whole or what it stands for.

TARGETING AND ORGANIZING NURSES

Historically, the American labor movement could not be called receptive to the needs of professionals (Lipset, 1967). In addition, professionals have not indicated an ideology reflective of commitment to the union movement. Professionals are concerned with their image, status, and the public transference of stereotypes of union members to their discipline and practice.

Though some unions made attempts to organize nurses prior to 1974, health care became a fertile area for union expansionist needs with the passage of the Taft-Hartley Amendments. The trade unions have been overt in stating their reasons for their departure from tradition in focusing their efforts on professionals and women. They are honest in saying they need to maintain their numbers to meet their members' needs. The corollary of this is that trade union leaders need to maintain their numbers so that they may retain their power and prestige within the political machinery of the labor movement.

The organizing drives that the author has witnessed can be best described as chauvinistic, paternalistic, patronizing, and most conspicuous in the absence of respect for educated, professional women. One unsuccessful attempt to organize nurses was described as "AFT's Million-Dollar Seduction Effort'' (Welch, 1979). It cannot be emphasized enough that trade union organizing drives are designed to capture one's emotional loyalty. Some of the more obvious methods employed include wining and dining or buying of potential converts and leafleting with flyers captioned with cliches such as "join the family" or "who will take care of the caretakers?" Major issues of controversy for the targeted groups will be identified and positions will be taken that sound supportive to either side. The literature published may or may not be factual.

In order to appeal to professionals, local unions will be developed exclusively for the group to provide an illusion of separation from the bulk of the membership. Professional nurses will be hired as organizers to create an image that nurses accept trade unionism. Fellow staff nurses may be receiving monies or even a salary above and beyond what they are earning as nurses to deliver the nurses' votes for the union. It is not an unusual procedure for trade unions to monetarily or materially reward those who deliver. These nurses serve as shills or Judas goats for their peers.*

The organizer will portray an image of power and militance, and make promises of improved economic and professional well-being. The organizer will also attempt to identify with personal characteristics such as race, minorities' needs, or soul power. Are nurses persuaded by the silvery bravado? In some instances, yes; in most, no.

When faced with the colorful and highly charged phrases and statements, the following questions should be considered:

1. Is the union membership favorable to the use of dues monies for wining and dining? Will dues money be used to provide services or will it be used to wine and dine others?

2. What is the rate of membership decline in the union? Will new membership enrollees serve merely to augment the needs of the other members?

3. Why are trade unions choosing the method of raiding already organized nursing groups? Is it because the "trade union pitch" is neither persuasive nor appealing to unorganized nurses?

4. Can one truly have a "professional union" affiliated with the AFL-CIO whose overwhelming membership is constituted from the crafts and industrial plants?

---

*Shills and Judas goats refer to nurses who organize for trade unions instead of professional organizations such as the state nurses associations. They support nonprofessional organizations or trade unions gaining control of nursing.

5. Why has the teachers' union targeted nurses when more than one million teachers are not represented for collective bargaining? Why have teachers preferred to join the National Education Association, whose membership outstrips the AFT by over one million?

6. How does the union justify the recent evidence that racial discrimination and practices continue in trade unions along with a willful neglect of rights and needs of minorities (Hill & Serrin, 1982)?

PROMISES AND POWER AND POLITICAL CLOUT

Nursing has been likened to a sleeping giant now ready to take the helm in decision making in the health care arena. Nurses want to have full professional status and to make a meaningful contribution; they are seeking the avenues and tools which will assist them in attaining the necessary clout to achieve their needs. Individual professional nurses are vulnerable. Nurses recognize what they desire but may not know where or how to go about getting it. For this reason, nurses may be easy prey for the polished, skillful trade union organizer who creates illusions and promises of power.

Labor has, to the objective observer, been described as suffering from malaise and an "inability to develop any persuasive appeal to white collar and professional employees" (Raskin, 1982, p. 1). But few nurses may be aware of this. Stereotypes created in the 1960s of powerful, militant organizations able to achieve their demands may well persist and yet become antiquated in the 1980s. Frequently during an organizing drive, one either does not have or does not take the time to research boasts of accomplishment. When successes are cited, ask when they were achieved; how they compared with organized and unorganized groups; and whether they were obtained by that trade union or was the union a part of a larger coalition of trade unions; and what were the givebacks? Malaise and power are antithetic to one another.

Real power is not limited to the workplace. If one is to be represented, one must have the ability to influence the positions and directions of the bargaining representative. The author believes that any local unit or local union of nurses will not have any power to influence their trade union representative. Sheer logic suggests that numbers determine the direction of action. If your bargaining unit is 5, 500, or 5,000, do you believe that you can influence a trade union whose membership is in the thousands? If your particular needs as a licensed professional conflict or differ from the bulk of the membership, is there really a chance of having them addressed? If the trade union takes positions that are counterproductive to your professional needs, will you be able to live with the knowledge that your dues support these movements?

Is there democracy in trade unions? Most of the literature suggests there is little. Aranowitz (1974, p. 412) states that, "on the whole, despite corruption and bureaucratic resistance to the exercise of membership control, many unions in the U.S. have retained the forms but not the content of democracy."

In a study of Local 1199, one of the unions representing nonprofessional health workers, it was well noted that democratic participation by membership was controlled and lacking and that the union itself mirrored other American unions as conservative stagnant bureaucracies (Ehrenreich, 1970). This union is one of labor's major contenders for professional nurses. Power is also noted to be at the national level. At the local level, you must consider what kind of understanding and reception you will receive from nonprofessionals or from another discipline? Will 1199 nurses be accepted and, if your bargaining outcomes are better than other members in the trade union, will you be ostracized or will you serve as a springboard for others to benefit from and possibly surpass? Even if your only concern is about power where you work, the union's agenda will have bearing in negotiations and grievances handling because they are concerned about their image and acceptability to the rest of their members and other trade unions.

Labor is suffering from its lack of political clout in today's world at all levels of government. The Teachers' Union in 1980 was extolling its political power to a group of nurses during an organizing drive in New York City. At the same time these promises were made, they had just lost their bid to obtain licensure for teachers in New York State. One is struck by the fact that professional nursing, which is perceived as lacking in power by trade unions, achieved licensure as early as 1903.

One must ask, are boasts of power real or imagined, and can non-nurse groups fulfill these promises for nurses? Won't the power of nurses and nursing be attenuated and diminished if we accede to the call of varied and competing trade unions and their interests?

An illusion is generally created that the trade union's political clout will be used to assist nurses in the legislative arena. In reality, nothing ever prevented, in the past or now, any of the unions from lending their support for nursing legislation; therefore, are they saying they will now turn their attention to nursing regulations if you vote for them? Will they guarantee that nursing legislation will be a part of their platform? What prevented them in the past from lending support and are they doing so now?

REPRESENTATION OF NURSES

Representation for the purposes of collective bargaining requires more than the skills of negotiation or knowledge of the law. Effective representation requires understanding of the industry, its history, customs, norms, rituals, and the nature of the work performed by the employee. Witness the difficulties the profession had in gaining acceptance and understanding for what nurses do from our colleagues in other health disciplines—can one then imagine that truck drivers, butchers, carpenters, or teachers will have greater insight? Wages and hours are but a small part—can you imagine these same individuals attempting to defend your grievances with respect to safe patient care, rotation, and nursing prerogatives? Will unions who represent nonprofessional health care workers aggressively defend your rights on nursing matters, especially if they're not in the best interests of the bulk of their membership? Labor relations is a political decision-making process, and many seemingly unrelated variables come into play when union members are agreeing to the outcomes.

Credibility is important to representation, not only for the group represented, but to external groups as well. How effective and knowledgeable do you think a non-nurse representative will be in developing demands and adjusting grievances? Even when the trade unions employ nurses, do you think that other people are unaware that it is non-nurses or nonprofessionals who hold the power and are issuing the orders?

The author, as a former faculty member, was represented by an affiliate of the AFT. It became clear at that time that the union not only could not, but would not, represent the needs of the nurse faculty. The nursing faculty noted with much chagrin that the school of nursing had less top-ranking and paying positions than did other academic departments; that the school had fewer tenured or job-secure positions; that the schedules and hours worked were more than professors in other departments; that the union would pay lip service and do nothing to help nurse faculty in the quest to receive equal pay for comparable worth or to achieve all the rights and privileges that academic colleagues in other departments had without question. In the event that a professor's contract was not renewed, the union could not even obtain for the individual the reasons for the termination. Though grievances regarding termination may have been filed, few were ever won. The school had for years been on the censure list of the professional association for university professors for violating the principles and rights of academic freedom, which is essential to any professor in the performance of his or her work. Did the union do anything? Did it make the reversal of this situation its top priority? It did not seem so. With respect to individual professional orientation, some nurse faculty were fearful of subtle retaliation if they took public positions of opposition to the parent union's attempts to organize nurses. What did this AFL-CIO professional union do? It protected the system, the high-paid senior tenured professors, the overwhelming majority of whom were men; it collected dues and functioned with an impotence that developed from a combination of governmental system bureaucracy and self-imposition. These experiences dramatically highlighted for this author the fact that trade union decisions were based first on what is good for the union, and second on what the whole membership wanted, and that concepts of professionalism were fantasy and illusion spoken about just to keep the troops in line. There was no concern for the particular needs of a licensed professional group as nurse faculty.

SOLIDARITY

Throughout nurses' education, the team approach and the importance of team cohesiveness was stressed. Recent evidence suggests that nurses believe that their power in a collective bargaining situation would be improved if the bargaining agent were the same for professional nurses, practical nurses, and nurses' aides (Beletz, 1980). On the other hand, many nurses share a belief that professional nurses' power would be diluted in this type of situation.

During an organizing drive, the power of numbers is stressed. Images are created that the entire trade union, if not the whole labor movement, will come to the support and defense of the demands of nurses. Rarely is mention made of the fact that support cannot be guaranteed, that support is determined by the politics of the moment, and that even when the bargaining agent is the same for multiple categories of personnel in the same institution, contracts covering these employees may expire at different times.

With respect to solidarity among different categories of employees, a fairly well known fact often forgotten during an organizing drive, is that one's economic, political, and professional orientation is strongly influenced by one's place in the industrial hierarchy, work position, and experiences (Lester, 1958).

In this respect, legal responsibility and accountability places the professional nurse in a position of directing and delegating to nonprofessionals various aspects of nursing care. The nature of the nurse's work, position, salary, and expectations as a professional affect the nurse's frame of reference and desires to be different from nonprofessionals. Since nonprofessionals outnumber the professionals, the outcome would be a diminution of nurses' power to influence the goals and objectives of the trade union.

The same would apply to nurses when they are members of an all-professional bargaining unit. It is more cost-effective for trade unions to bargain and service one group of professionals than it is to have a singular subgroup of professional nurses. At this time, it has been determined that nurses have a sufficiently different community of interest from other professionals, so that they are allowed to have a separate bargaining unit. Since trade unions are businesses which are economically hurting, it would not be unreasonable for them to institute cost-saving measures by both encouraging and supporting an elimination of single units for nurses.

Of course, during an organizing drive a trade union would refute these cited loopholes in their solidarity argument. However, you should then ask what guarantees will be made so that the particular interests and needs of nurses will be advanced, regardless of the desires of all the trade union's non-nurse members? Can these guarantees be had in writing? Since it is difficult to rid oneself of a trade union once it is voted in, what assurance would be given that the trade union would not reverse its position at some point in the future?

One other point about power. A trade union wins an election when a majority of those voting vote for them. Trade union representation is, and has always been, very controversial in nursing. In one study, a majority of nurses were in opposition to an affiliation with traditional organized labor unions such as the AFL-CIO (Beletz, 1980). If a trade union wins by a very small majority, chances are that many nurses will not be supportive of the trade union, and will not follow its directions, thereby markedly reducing the power the union seeks to project. There is a difference between winning a battle and winning a war.

PROFESSIONALISM AND TRADE UNION COMPATIBILITY

The hallmark of a true profession has always been the right of self-governance. It is the public which grants this right in return for which the profession, in a trust relationship, determines and maintains standards and quality practice. The right of self-governance necessitates that the profession speak for itself. Intrinsic to nursing has been the following continued observation:

> There still persists too great a lack of "professional identity" among nurses, large pockets of professional property, and a wide gap between the group of nurses who want professional freedom and autonomy "right now" and the group who are fearful of and intimidated by this social growth. (Driscoll, 1967)

Nurse freedom, autonomy, and power are today's watchwords. These concepts are alluring and desired, and rightfully so. The nurse also is frequently unsophisticated in the techniques of organizing and will fall prey as these concepts are capitalized on. Some nurses are beguiled by the organizer's antics and seek a Lancelot to protect their dreams.

In reality, the price that the individual nurse—and the collective of the profession—pays for trade union representation is exorbitant and untenable. Forfeited are nurses' rights to determine their own destiny; to control their practice, working conditions, and professional affairs; to advance their particular needs; to speak for and represent themselves; to be perceived as an untainted profession by the many publics nurses interact with. Nursing history is replete with attempts by various groups seeking to control the profession. Nursing is the heart of the health delivery system. Trade union representation destroys nurses' unique professional identity and renders them pawns designated to provide the adrenalin for the economically hurting trade union movement. Ultimately, trade unions are not protectors, but serve as predators of nurses' rights and this, therefore, renders trade unionism incompatible with nursing professionalism. In addition, the previously cited lack of concern for the needs of professionals, women, and minorities, the lack of democracy, the diminished power and clout, and the inability to achieve concessions at the bargaining table renders any nurse who votes for a trade union beholden to a chauvinistic, ailing, and antiquated bureaucracy.

Ultimately, a profession is not a trade. Professional nurse power will only be achieved through a commitment to one another, and a solidarity of purpose with the goals of the profession. Trade union representation does not provide power. If anything, it dilutes, diminishes, and may destroy the nurse power because it fragments, is divisive, and creates discourse for the profession and confusion for the public.

REFERENCES

Aranowitz, S. Trade unionism in America. In B. Silverman, & M. Yanowich, (Eds.), *The worker in "post industrial" capitalism*. New York: The Free Press, 1974, p. 412.

Beletz, E. E. Organized nurses view their collective bargaining agent. *Supervisor Nurse: Journal for Nursing Leadership and Management*, September, 1980, 11, 45.

Driscoll, V. M. A decade of action and of growth. *The New York State Nurse*, August 1967, 39, 3.

Ehrenreich, J. Local 1199: Where is it leading? *Health PAC Bulletin*, July-August 1970, 22, 15.

General Shoe Company. National Labor Relations Board (NLRB), *77*, 124, 127 (1948).

Getman, J., Goldberg, S. B., & Herman, J. B. N.L.R.B. regulation of campaign tactics: The behavioral assumptions on which the board regulates. *Stanford Law Review*, July 1975, *27*, 1465–1492.

Hill, H. Labor's enemy labor. *New York Times*, September 5, 1982, p. E17.

Hill, H., & Serrin, W. Study finds racial discrimination persists in U.S. labor movement. *New York Times Sunday*, June 6, 1982, p. 16y.

Lester, R. A. *As unions mature*. Princeton, N.J.: Princeton University Press, 1958.

Lipset, S. M. White collar workers and professionals—Their attitudes and behaviors toward unions. In W. A. Faunce (Ed.), *Readings in Industrial Sociology*. New York: Appleton-Century-Crofts, 1967.

Raskin, A. H. Frustrated and wary labor marks its day. *New York Times Sunday*, September 5, 1982, p. 1; 6F.

Rees, A. *The economics of trade unions*, (2nd ed., rev.). Chicago: University of Chicago Press, 1977.

Welch, C. A. Editorial: A.F.T.'s million-dollar seduction effort. *The Journal of the New York State Nurses' Association*, August 1979, *10*, 5.

Part II

THEORETICAL STUDIES AND RESPONSES

Part II contains five research studies and five respondents' comments/critiques of the studies. The first study is ''The Power of Nursing's Leader Elite.'' It is the first part of a planned three-phase study to assess the continuing educational needs of nurses in advanced roles. This study attempted to identify the learning needs of graduate-prepared nurses in leadership positions by analyzing their report of critical incidents to their enactment of the leadership role. The population studied were nurse educators in basic, graduate, continuing, or inservice nursing education programs; administrators of such programs; and administrators or supervisors of hospital or community health agency nursing services. A mailed questionnaire was sent to selected nurse leaders in a 50-mile radius from New York City. The instrument was designed to contain two effective and two ineffective situations (critical incidents). The findings of the study should be reviewed within the framework of a low return rate (10.2 percent) and the exploratory nature of the first phase of a study.

The response to the study on ''The Power of Nursing's Leader Elite'' focused on the inherent difficulties in the design employed in the study and the low response rate to the questionnaire containing the critical incidents. It is important in nursing—in terms of power—to consider the fact that subjects reported twice as many ineffective incidents as effective ones. Three findings are of interest and will be looked at in the second phase of the study. They were the identification of ineffective patterns of communication, ineffective evaluation of performance, and the anger expressed by nursing leader elite. According to Frederickson (Chapter 7, Response), the implications for both power and politics are the "heart of the nursing profession today." The results of the studies were viewed by the respondent through a psychological-developmental framework. Frederickson also suggests that the researcher use marketing techniques to improve the return on her research questionnaire in phases two and three of the planned project.

"The Academic Power of Nursing Deans" is the second research study presented in this book. It was completed by a researcher who is currently a chairperson of a department of nursing at a state university. The purpose of this study was to analyze the relationship between the processes of socialization experienced prior to assumption of the decanal role and the demands of that role. The aspects of socialization addressed were age, education, and role preparation. Age was studied in order to learn whether it had any relationship to the deans' perception of power. Education was studied because it was anticipated that deans with a high level of academic preparation for the role would perceive of themselves as having a high degree of role power. Role-preparation was the third variable studied because subjects who had attended specific programs of learning directly related to the decanal role or who held prior dean positions would view themselves as being high in role power. Dean and power were defined for the study. The six functional areas used as indices for power measurement were: university affairs, budget, faculty, students, curriculum, and professional affairs. A two-part questionnaire was used for data collection. The response rate was 78.5 percent of the potential subjects selected for the study who met the criteria outlined by the researcher. The findings indicated that, as a group, deans of nursing do not see themselves as having a high degree of role power. Deans of nursing see themselves as having the same amount of role power as deans who are their counterparts and the researcher found that there was no significant relationship between any of the socialization factors studied and the perceptions of power held by deans of nursing. There was a discussion in this study of the fact that deans of nursing are predominantly females in a role within the university that has been traditionally male. This may or may not have influenced the power associated with the decanal role. It certainly makes sense that in the nursing profession, which is predominantly female, deans of nursing should also predominantly be female.

McGriff was the respondent to the investigation "The Academic Power of Nursing Deans." She found the definitions employed in the previous study to be too restrictive, and she backs up her opinions with interesting facts. McGriff was at the time a director of a division of nursing in a private university in New York City, and she was well qualified to critique the study. An interesting point to study in the future would be the relationship of the power concept of deans of nursing to the politics in the university/college setting and to the input the dean of nursing has on university policy. McGriff thinks that deans of nursing should have knowledge and academic preparation in nursing, administration, and higher education.

The third research study in this section is a field study to explore the policy making process in the state of Florida on a proposed amendment to the Florida Nurse Practice Act. Mixon attempted to study in the late 1970s a topic that has implications in many states in the 1980s and for planning in the 1990s. "Public Policy Making on a Nursing Issue" is a systematic examination of how public policy is determined on a nursing issue at the state level on proposed legislation which directly would impact on the practice of nursing. Data collection consisted of interviews with the key participants on the amendment to analyze the policy process, the study of minutes and written reports and documents dealing with the legislation, and the researcher's personal observations of state committee deliberations on the proposed legislative measures. A senator from the state of Florida initiated and sponsored Senate Bill 1038 which would affect the Florida Nurse Practice Act. He hoped it would control the high cost of health care services in the state. There were three provisions of S.B. 1038. These were: to amend the definition of the practice of professional nursing by deleting an advisory committee and authorizing the board of nursing to decide what constitutes advanced and specialized levels of nursing practice; to allow for third-party reimbursement for nursing care and thereby encourage independent nursing private practices; and to require that the Department of Health and Rehabilitative Services make available to eligible Medicaid recipients the services of a certified advanced registered nurse practitioner. The bill failed to pass on a 3 to 3 tie vote. Perhaps the most fascinating part of this field study was the descriptions by the investigator of the players in the government and those representing professional nursing. This study focuses not only on policy but just as much on politics and the power in nursing and state governments.

The response to "Public Policy Making on a Nursing Issue" focused on the use of Dye's model to describe and explore the causes and consequences of governmental activity as a means of understanding public policy. Natapoff points out that the researcher did not explicitly outline Dye's framework for analysis; it nevertheless, in her opinion, should be identified. The model requires the content of policy to be outlined, the impact of environmental forces to be analyzed, institutional arrangements to be studied, the results of political processes on policy formulation to be analyzed, and the consequences of the policy on society to be evaluated. Mixon's study is heavy on the first several steps in Dye's model and lighter on the last few. This is perhaps an area where further research should be done. It is important that nurses pay attention to Mixon's study and Natapoff's response because in several states there are legislative bills proposed to amend the Nurse Practice Act. Other researchers should use either the field study approach and/or Dye's framework to gather data about the public policy making process in their own state.

"Dilemmas in Decision Making" is a study about nursing input into the decision-making process in the health care arena, "to gain and yield power effectively." Blagman's study involved patient care decisions made by staff nurses in the hospital setting. She addressed three variables: values/utility; risk-taking behaviors; and personality characteristics. The relationships studied were: the nurses' level of educational preparation for nursing practice; the number of years of nursing experience; and the modality (e.g. primary nursing) of nursing care in the institutions studied; the research decision-maker variables concerning alternatives of a specific decision situation; and situational variables. The subjects in the study were from eight New York metropolitan area hospitals. There were 97 females and one male staff nurse studied. The editor believes the male probably should have been removed from the study. The Edwards Personal Preference Schedule was used by Blagman for personality data collection. Values and risk-taking behaviors were studied by the Kogan-Wallach Choice Dilemma Questionnaire. Ten nursing dilemmas were also conducted by the investigator which involved nursing care decisions for immobilized patients. The researcher chose immobilized patient care situations because it is a commonplace nursing problem in the acute care setting. The findings in this study indicated staff nurses were neither cautious nor risky. Their personality characteristics were stronger in the personal caring aspects of their jobs as such nurturance behavior, but lacked enough strength in the more powerful characteristics of their personalities. Nurses in this study needed to have a stronger sense of autonomy in practice and assertiveness in the work environment. Unfortunately, Blagman's study did not indicate that staff nurses had input into major patient care decisions in the traditional administrative model. Therefore they had a feeling of powerlessness. Blagman thinks that when decision making is decentralized, staff nurses will have more power in the decision-making situation in the services they give to patients and families. It would be hard to disagree with Blagman's analysis that having more power over staffing ratios, standards of care, and staff development will yield more personal power for nurses.

The response to "Dilemmas in Decision Making" focused on what can be done in the nursing curriculum and the service setting to create a more positive environment for improving risk-taking behaviors of beginning staff nurses. The preceptor program concept was explored as a method by which, O'Leary believes, the senior level student has an opportunity for the decision making process to be experiential rather than theoretical. She further believes that merging the needs of education and nursing practice together would decrease "reality shock," which is frequently associated with the first job in one's profession. Modalities of nursing care are also reviewed. Primary nursing is the method in which nurses are responsible for their own practice decisions for a 24-hour period. Nurses are then accountable to patients and peers, to professional organizations, and to the courts for their professional conduct. This yields more autonomy in practice and more personal power in the acute care setting for staff nurses.

"Organized Nurses and Collective Bargaining: Opinions, Participation, and Militance" is the fifth study in Part II. It is an investigation into the collective bargaining practices in the nursing profession. This study by Beletz deals with probably one of the most controversial practices in nursing today. The topic itself can generate much emotionalism and misconceptions which obviously color one's reaction and ability to deal with and conduct research into the area. This investigation is the longest in the book because of the highly controversial nature of the topic, the lack of good research in the area, and the need to provide background information and history about collective bargaining. Collective bargaining began in the 1960s in nursing. Basically, it started as a means to achieve objectives in the work environment in the hospital setting in a timely fashion. Many directors of nursing or vice presidents for nursing lack the power in the hospital to bring about changes in nursing employment in their hospitals. At first, collective bargaining was used to gain salary increases and the assignment of non-nursing tasks to other hospital workers. Strikes were not mentioned in contracts 20 years ago. Times have changed, societal values toward unionism have changed, strikes do occur, and collective bargaining is used as a collective weapon to obtain more acceptable working relationships and environments in the hospital setting. Many state nurses' associations have organized nurses in the health care industry. Nurses in both the hospital and community setting are represented by their professional organization for collective bargaining purposes. Nurses in the educational arena are represented more frequently by nonprofessional unions. Some nurse educators belong to the union which represents their college and/or university and a state nurses' association. Collective bargaining is a means of distribution of power within the employment setting. It helps nurses achieve more power, autonomy, and control over practice in the clinical setting. The contract can be viewed as the basis of labor-management relationships and the process of agreement between the institution and professional nurses. The bargaining process and the resultant agreement impact upon the nurses private and professional life. Beletz's study focused on the relationship between perceptions of collective bargaining, participation in collective bargaining, and selected demographic variables among nurses employed in voluntary hospitals in New York state that are represented by the State Nurses Association for collective bargaining purposes. New York State and New York State Nurses Association (NYSNA) was chosen because NYSNA is the largest recognized collective bargaining agent for nurses in the United States. The research methodology employed was a descriptive survey utilizing a mailed questionnaire. The response rate was 58 percent. The tool was piloted for reliability and clarity of items. The findings indicated that perceptions of collective bargaining were associated with geographic location, basic nursing preparation, year of graduation from basic nursing program, and age. Advantages of the bargaining process correlated with experience/years subjects had used collective bargaining, geographic location, and race. Perception of power in relationship to the bargaining agent was identified by geographic location and the year of graduation from the subjects' basic nursing program. The professional model of collective bargaining correlated with geographic location, basic preparation for practice, year of graduation from basic program, age, race, sex, and position. The union model was associated with basic nursing preparation, race, and position in the hospital. Participation in collective bargaining correlated with the number of years of continuous practice, position in the hospital, and number of years organized for collective bargaining purposes in addition to the nurses' having voted in the positive for the bargaining agent. Militance was associated with age, race, religion, basic nursing education, year of graduation from basic program, years of continuous practice, membership in the Association prior to collective bargaining, and geographic location. These findings are also described in tabular form.

The respondent to "Organized Nurses and Collective Bargaining: Opinions, Participation, and Militance" focused on the fact that this was the first study limited exclusively to nurses organized for collective bargaining purposes and that further research needs to be done on the same topic in other states and even repeated in New York in the 1980s. It will be interesting for researchers to study trends in collective bargaining in the 1980s in nursing. This is a time when the health care industry is being asked to be cost-effective and the reimbursement payment policies in hospitals are being changed dramatically. Nursing has done well in the 1970s and early 1980s in New York through the collective bargaining process represented by New York State Nurses Association. The question to ask for this State Association and for others is, can they maintain the power they have achieved and move forward? Wieczorek, in her response, believes that collective bargaining is here to stay in nursing in the health care arena. As jobs in nursing become harder to find, more nurses will organize for collective bargaining purposes. According to new items in the American Journal of Nursing, there are many states in which there are no open positions for nurses in the hospital. This has great importance in the profession when one considers that about 80 percent of the nurses in this country are employed in the hospital setting. Perhaps nurses will gain more power in the system in the 1980s. In order to accomplish this, nurses need to make known to everyone that they are worth the cost of their services. This can be facilitated through the power of the collective bargaining process.

[7]

Continuing Education: The Power of Nursing's Leader Elite

Andrea B. O'Connor

INTRODUCTION

Spiraling health care costs, quality of health care services, access to health care services, and questions surrounding the issues of shortages and/or oversupply of various types of health personnel are topics debated by hospital administrators, politicians, nurses, physicians, and other groups. The media frequently plays on the heart strings of the public when it comes to the subject of the treatment of acute illness, chronic disease, and hospitalization. The public is often confused and frightened of the health care delivery system and its professional personnel.

Nursing is a sleeping giant in the health care delivery industry. The sheer numbers, knowledge, and skills of nurses have never been effectively harnessed for utilization of power within the system and with the recipients of the system's services—the consumers. Nursing leadership development is needed to meet the challenges posed in a changing technological society. Nurses can learn to use power and apply effective political strategies to bring about health policy changes that will impact positively on the health care system and consumer satisfaction. A method of achieving this is the continuing education program for nursing's leader elite.

STATISTICS OF NURSING'S LEADER ELITE

There are 1,027,307 employed registered nurses in the United States and of this number, approximately 8 percent have master's or doctoral degrees ("Survey Shows a Million RNs Employed," 1980). The majority of nurses with advanced education are in leadership positions in health care facilities, higher educational institutions, government, professional societies, and the publishing industry where they try to facilitate, improve, and direct the care provided by other nurses with less preparation. Little attention has been directed to identifying the best ways to educate nurse leaders for the roles they will assume or to provide for their continued learning once they are practicing in more advanced roles. Yet, if the nursing profession is to advance its ability to provide high quality health care, the capacity of the profession's leadership to guide and direct that advance must be ensured. This is a role for continuing professional education for nursing's leader elite.

The educational needs of nurse leaders employed in educational and administrative roles are varied and complex. This study represents the first systematic assessment of the continuing educational needs of nurses in advanced roles. It attempted to identify the learning needs of graduate-prepared nurses in leadership positions by analyzing their report of critical incidents to their enactment of the leadership role.

METHODOLOGY

In this study, nurse leaders were defined as nurses prepared at the graduate (master's or doctoral) level whose primary positions were those of educators in basic, graduate, continuing, or inservice nursing education programs; administrators of such programs; and administrators or supervisors of hospital or community health agency nursing services. Clinical nurse specialists prepared at the graduate level were included if their job responsibilities involved staff education and/or supervisory functions.

The sample was drawn from a 50-mile radius of New York City. It included nurse leaders employed in National League for Nursing-accredited nursing programs offering associate degree, baccalaureate degree, or graduate level education in nursing; Joint Commission on Accreditation of Hospitals-accredited hospitals with a bed capacity of 200 or more; and community health agencies offering nursing services endorsed by the Home Health Assembly of New Jersey, the Home Care Association of New York State, or the Association of Community

Health Service Agencies, Inc. (Connecticut). The sample was therefore drawn from a three-state geographic area which met the characteristics described previously.

INSTRUMENTATION

A central theme in adult education is the assessment of the adult learners' needs. Knowles (1970) describes superior adult learning conditions. He identified the three following areas necessary for learning to take place: (1) the learner feels the need to learn; (2) the learner espouses the goals of learning as his own goals; (3) the learner shares responsibility for planning and implementing the learning experience. Successful educational programming depends on the prior identification of learning needs as a basis for educational program planning.

Despite its importance to the adult education marketplace, the concept of need is not clearly defined in the adult education literature (Monett, 1977). A variety of different approaches currently exist to assess the educational needs of the learner. These multiple types of assessments are based on input from a variety of different sources. Most authorities recommend the use of several approaches to delineate between individual learners' felt and real continuing educational needs: to incorporate the needs of the employing organization/institution; to incorporate the larger society; and to select priorities and establish goals as a data base for program planning (Knowles, 1970; Lorig, 1977; Bell, 1978).

This investigation was designed to be the first part of a three-phase educational needs assessment study, each phase expected to verify and build upon data collected in prior phases.

The critical incident technique was chosen for this study. It is a job analysis approach to needs assessment (Bell, 1978) that obtains learner input within a context that permits analysis of organizational and societal as well as individual educational needs. The concerns of all three groups were included because collectively they have a stake in the outcome of the final program content. Both the learner (by reporting the incidents) and the educator (through data analysis) thus contribute to the identification of learning needs.

The critical incident research technique is a systematic method for recording, analyzing, and synthesizing observed behaviors to yield the critical requirements of an activity (Flanagan, 1954). The technique has been used in diverse areas of nursing research related to the topic of the investigation. Other studies using this technique have included the identification of learning needs (Malfetti, 1955), and the analysis of leadership behaviors of head nurses, supervisors, and directors in hospital settings (Hagen & Wolff, 1961).

A mailed questionnaire was sent to nurse leaders. They were asked to describe behaviors in actual real situations in which they felt particularly effective or ineffective in some aspect of their leadership role. Subjects were asked to report on two effective and two ineffective situations.

FINDINGS

One hundred and thirty-two nurse leaders reported 589 usable critical incidents. The mailed questionnaire resulted in a 10.2 percent response rate. Not all respondents reported four incidents, but several of the incident reports contained more than one critical behavior, and these were treated by the investigator as separate critical incidents. The incidents reported were subdivided into two basic categories: 312 (53 percent) involved effective behaviors and 277 (47 percent), ineffective behaviors. The findings of the study should be considered within the framework of a low return rate, and the exploratory nature of the study. There was, however, the provision for follow-up in future phases of the project to verify the findings using a second and third needs assessment approach. No novel incidents were encountered in the second half of the questionnaires analyzed. This suggests that the findings do identify some of the learning needs of nursing leaders.

The majority of respondents (68, or 52 percent) were employed in hospitals at the time of the study; 42 (32 percent) held positions in colleges or universities; 13 (10 percent) held positions in home health agencies; and 9 (7 percent) failed to identify their place of employment. Position titles reported by respondents were nursing education organization executive (dean or program director) (62 percent); professor (25 percent); continuing education/staff development instructor (10 percent); supervisor or clinical coordinator (12 percent); nursing organization executive (26 percent); clinical specialist (8 percent); and other or no response (8 percent). Eighty percent reported a master's degree as their highest educational preparation; 3 percent were doctorally-prepared.

All critical incidents were coded and then abstracted using the following method: the role and subrole, if any, of the reporter was identified; the role partner or partners were identified; the setting in which the incident occurred was identified; key phrases in the incident report descriptive of the critical behavior were underlined; and a brief statement summarizing the critical behavior was written. Reliability of the abstracting procedure was established by having two nurse researchers familiar with the technique employed to abstract independently 55 random incidents. Reliability estimates were computed using an agreement-disagreement formula (Fine et al., 1965). A reliability of 0.85 was obtained. After completion of the abstracting procedure, each summary statement was placed on an individual file card for further analysis.

While the incident reports themselves are a rich source of information concerning the learning needs of nurse leaders, their level of specificity limits the application of findings to policy and programming decisions. Therefore, a means of organizing the data base to provide a general view of leader behaviors suggestive of learning needs is necessary. This organization seeks to preserve the distinct behaviors addressed in the incidents while offering a framework within which these behaviors can be described.

The investigator chose an inductive approach to organize the data for analysis. Using this approach, the incidents were grouped on commonalities in reported behaviors. As broad categories emerged, they were tentatively labeled. Where appropriate, subcategories that further clarified aspects of the broad categories were identified using the same approach. The deductive approach—using a preselected framework for analysis and sorting the incidents into established categories—was rejected as being unsuited to the purposes of the study. Deductive analysis tends to produce convergent, and hence conventional, solutions. An exploration of leaders' learning needs seemed to demand an analysis that would permit emergence of unusual, unsuspected categories of behavior.

Two nurse leaders participated in an assessment of the categorization of incidents as a reasonable way of organizing the data. Using an agreement-disagreement formula, a reliability of .88 was achieved for the broad categories, and .80 for the subcategories.

IDENTIFIED CATEGORIES

The category containing the largest number of incidents, 28 percent of the total, reflected behaviors related to *Communication Skills*. Stated positively, Communication Skills involved such activities as providing relevant information in a rational manner, clarifying and explaining, listening, and setting a climate that facilitates communication. Of incidents in this category, 54 percent were reported as ineffective. Ineffective behaviors involved failing to control anger or frustration, failing to confront another when a problem arises, failing to act assertively to achieve goals, failing to explore reasons for another's position, and failing to focus on the issues.

The second largest category, containing 16 percent of the incidents, was *Performance Evaluation*. Incidents in this category involved the evaluation of behaviors of nursing staff members, non-nurse subordinates, and students. Behaviors indicative of this category included: establishing performance standards; documenting and communicating performance deficits; planning for improved performance; and following norms and procedures related to the evaluation process. Ineffective incidents were reported twice as often as were effective incidents. Ineffective behaviors involved failing to clarify expectations for performance, failing to communicate performance deficits, allowing anger to interfere with the evaluation, failing to follow up, and failing to maintain confidentiality.

Management Practices was the third largest category, containing 11 percent of incidents. Ineffective incidents were slightly more frequent than were effective incidents in this category. Behaviors related to a full range of administrative activities, including planning, policy determination and implementation, maintenance of positive intraorganizational relationships, office management, time management, and resource acquisition, allocation, and training. Ineffective Management Practices included failure to obtain information needed for job performance, the hiring of unqualified candidates for a particular position, failure to delegate appropriately or to use time effectively, and inability to influence others to accept a decision.

Teaching Practices contained 11 percent of the incidents. Eighty-two percent of incidents were reported as effective. Teaching Practices included incidents related to content selection, such as basing content on a needs assessment of learners' knowledge or experience, and the process of teaching, such as selecting teaching strategies and creating an environment for learning. Teaching Practices reported in these incidents involved both students and staff members as learners. The few ineffective behaviors reported in this category involved instances where the teacher took over an activity from a learner, which detracted from the learning experience, and where the teacher failed to prevent or halt disruptive behaviors in the classroom or clinical setting.

Conflict Management contained 7 percent of incidents, and included behaviors related to the use of various conflict resolution strategies in conflicts involving oneself or others. Forty percent of these incidents were reported as ineffective; they represented difficulties in assessing the conflict situation before attempting to intervene and failure to structure the environment, for example, by moving conflicting parties away from the patient's bedside or other public place.

Problem Solving also accounted for 7 percent of the incidents, with 90 percent in this category reflecting effective behaviors. Problem Solving behaviors involved individual efforts to identify and use resources or to act directly in solving a problem, as well as behaviors engaging others in problem-solving activities. The few ineffective behaviors in this category related to failure to clarify the nature of the problem and failure to facilitate others' use of problem-solving strategies.

Incidents related to *Self Esteem* represented 5 percent of the total, with the majority categorized as ineffective. These incidents involved the respondent's report of feelings of inadequacy concerning knowledge and/or skills, job performance, reactions to criticism, and ability to cope with stress.

The category *Change Process* contained 5 percent of incidents, about equally divided between effective and ineffective behaviors. This category involved various phases of introducing, implementing, and evaluating a planned change. Ineffective behaviors centered on aspects of assessment, such as determining how others are reacting to plans, establishing groundwork, and selecting an optimum time to introduce a change; working out the mechanics of a change; and planning for and conducting follow-up activities to evaluate and sustain the change.

Political Savvy accounted for 4 percent of behaviors, again equally divided between effective and ineffective behaviors. Political Savvy involved developing and implementing a political strategy to achieve goals. Ineffective behaviors centered around the inability to influence peers and the inability to recognize informal rules operating in a given situation.

Nursing Intervention contained 3 percent of the reported incidents, with twice as many effective as ineffective behaviors. Behaviors in this category involved interactions with or on the behalf of patients' families as well as patients themselves. Respondents frequently identified their role as patient advocate. Ineffective behaviors in this category tended to reflect an inability to achieve desired patient care goals.

Behaviors related to the use of *Group Process* accounted for 3 percent of the total incidents. Incidents in this category were overwhelmingly effective, and related to the use of the group process to complete a task, facilitate communications, negotiate, and identify and address others' concerns.

Role Modeling was contained in 1 percent of the incidents. Incidents in this category reported the use of role modeling to train subordinates in management techniques—particularly labor negotiation strategies—and to teach patient advocacy and assertiveness behaviors. Ineffective incidents involved a failure to adequately model the behavior being formally taught.

The final category, *Crisis Intervention*, contained 1 percent of the incidents, which were almost all effective. These incidents involved intervention to resolve a clinical crisis situation or to facilitate another's management of a personal or professional crisis.

QUALITATIVE VERSUS QUANTITATIVE

Numbers provide a convenient means of summarizing findings and pointing to key areas of concern. Quantitative results in this study should be viewed with caution. Emphasis should be placed on the qualitative findings.

The question posed to respondents to stimulate their report of incidents was made deliberately general by the investigator to elicit a broad range of incidents occurring in a variety of settings and involving both formal employment and other professional activities. This deliberate lack of focus on specific activities coupled with the different positions held by respondents meant that novel situations were likely to emerge, representing important learning needs, but not appearing in large numbers. This factor coupled with the low response rate to the questionnaire meant that a single category of behavior may be of great importance even though it contains only a few incidents. A follow-up study using a different needs assessment approach would be necessary to quantify needs as a means of prioritizing them for program planning.

The same caution should be applied in considering the effective versus ineffective behaviors. Both classes should be examined in determining learning needs. While ineffective behaviors clearly suggest learning needs, behaviors in a single category may be both effective and ineffective. Indeed, some respondents reported both effective and ineffective behaviors related to a single aspect of role, suggesting a focus on one type of activity performed effectively at some times and ineffectively at others.

FINDINGS RELATED TO POWER, POLITICS, AND POLICY

Claus and Bailey (1977) view leadership as a multidimensional phenomenon involving the use of power through managerial functions and human relations processes to influence the behavior of others to achieve specified goals. Their Power/Authority/Influence Leadership Model provides a good framework for examining study findings as they relate to power, politics, and policy.

In the Power/Authority/Influence model, authority derives from the leader's power bases—personal, organizational, and social. Power is defined as strength, rooted in a positive self-concept, energy, and action. The identification of *Self-Esteem* as a category of leader behaviors fits into this aspect of the model. The preponderance of ineffective incidents in this category, reflecting low self-esteem, suggests a possible source of powerlessness among nurses in positions of leadership. Organizational power, in the form of positional authority, may be insufficient to overcome the effects of low self-esteem.

According to this model, authority—derived from the leader's power —gives rise to specific actions to reach identified goals. These actions involve both managerial functions and human relations processes that seek to influence others to act. Most of the behavioral categories identified in the study can be labeled as most closely related to either managerial functions or human relations processes. Together, these behaviors are the means to achieve political goals.

The categories *Management Practices, Performance Evaluation, Change Process*, and to a lesser extent, *Teaching Practices* and *Nursing Intervention*, represent leadership behaviors designed to establish a climate for action and provide resources for action to occur. In the incident reports, ineffective behaviors related to management functions included problems with planning, delegating, clarifying expectations, making decisions, providing for follow-up and documentation, acquiring resources, and communicating in a clear, timely, and dispassionate manner. These behaviors pervade all aspects of management for effective action, and necessarily affect the leader's power to influence others to achieve goals.

The use of *Group Process, Problem Solving, Conflict Management*, and *Crisis Intervention* are human relations activities that help others move toward goals. The incident reports suggest that nurse leaders are more skilled in these aspects of leadership function. Fewer ineffective incidents appear in categories representing human relations processes than in those related to management functions.

Influence is accomplished through behaviors categorized in this study as *Political Savvy* and *Role Modeling*. Incidents in these categories suggest some difficulties in planning political strategies, assessing the climate for action, convincing others to act, and modeling effective behaviors.

Overriding all of these activities is the need for *Communication Skills* to express power as authority, set in motion needed management functions, effectively intervene to promote sound human relations, and influence others to action. Kalisch and Kalisch (1982), among others, stress the relational nature of power. Power cannot exist in a vacuum, and it requires two or more interacting people. Politics, too, is a relational process, as two or more people compete for scarce resources (Kalisch & Kalisch, 1982). Such interactions necessarily involve communication skills, which Stevens (1981) identifies as a key need for leaders. *Communication Skills* was the category containing most of the incidents reported by nurse leaders. Similar behaviors also appeared in other categories, although in more specific contexts. Time and time again, leaders reported incidents related to anger, and the effects control or lack of control of anger and frustration had on the leader's ability to act effectively to achieve a goal. One must wonder why nurse leaders are so angry and what effect anger has had on the profession's power to achieve its political goals.

IMPLICATIONS

Findings of this study suggest several policy concerns related to the education and utilization of nursing leaders. First, how can we best educate nurses at the undergraduate and graduate levels to assume leadership roles? What skills do the incidents suggest are needed for effective leadership? When this study was undertaken, the investigator anticipated that incidents would reflect learning needs related to specific skills needed to perform a job, such as budget planning, teaching strategies, public speaking, preparation of reports and documents. The investigator hoped to elicit incidents reflecting other aspects of the leader's role related to authority and influence.

The incident reports suggest a need for a blend of practical skills to enable the leader to perform in a position plus human relations skills to promote effective interactions among others to achieve goals. Effective interactions with others require practice and experience. Therefore, one way of teaching the communications and human relations skills identified in this study would be to provide ample and varied opportunities for practicing these behaviors and analyzing outcomes. This experience would yield concrete information to the learner for use in her work situation.

While the incident report did not elicit identification of alternative solutions to the problem reported, many respondents speculated on the incident and what they might have handled differently in order to be more effective. In this investigation, nurse leaders seemed unable to identify more than one approach to managing a problematic situation. This possibility should be investigated in future research, but the evidence of this study indicates that nursing education should work to promote creative thinking among potential leaders, provoking the generation of multiple solutions to problems and the critique of their utility and consequences. Growth and change in the profession are impossible if nurses remain unwilling and unable to innovate.

A second concern raised by the study is how best to facilitate leadership development among emergent nurse leaders. What situations and relationships tend to thwart effective leader behavior, and how can these be managed to build leaders?

Analysis of the setting of the incidents is incomplete. However, inspection of the data reported indicates that many incidents occurred in office settings, at meetings, and in the clinical area. Nurse leaders tend to learn leadership behaviors in highly structured classroom settings. Transfer to the more typical environments in which they function may be more difficult to achieve. Role playing and other educational strategies that promote the transfer process of learning should be incorporated in programs of leader education.

Interactions with nurse superiors were far more likely to be ineffective than were those with other role partners. Least problematic were interactions with clients (students, patients). This suggests a need to deal with authority issues and relationships in preparing nurses for leadership roles. Nurse leaders in top positions should also recognize the potential for faulty interactions as viewed by subordinates, and they should take steps to clarify the communication process and explore difficulties as a means of promoting leadership development in subordinates.

Role modeling also was identified as a leader behavior useful in teaching subordinates how to perform specific job-related skills. This type of activity can probably be used to good effect in both on-the-job training and in formal leadership development programs.

A third policy consideration is the formulation of continuing education programs to promote the continued growth and development of nursing's leader elite. While verification of study findings should be conducted to further clarify and prioritize leaders' learning needs, results point to a program of nursing leadership development through continuing education that addresses the specific practice skills needed by nurses in specific leadership roles using teaching strategies that promote the development of interactional skills useful in all leadership functions. This suggests a curricular approach to professional continuing education for nursing leaders that contains themes related to the development of those skills that will enhance the power and political savvy of nurses so that they can perform effectively in their roles for the self-advancement and that of the profession.

REFERENCES

Bell, D. F. Assessing educational needs: Advantages and disadvantages of eighteen techniques. *Nurse Educator*, 1978, 3(5), 15–21.
Claus, K. E., & Bailey, J. T. *Power and influence in health care: A new approach to leadership*. St. Louis: C. V. Mosby, 1977.
Fine, J. L.; Malfetti, J. L.; & Shoben, E. J. *The development of a criterion for driver education*. New York: Teachers College Press, 1965.
Flanagan, J. C. The critical incident technique. *Psychological Bulletin*, 1954, 51, 327–358.
Hagen, E., & Wolff, L. *Nursing leadership behavior in general hospitals*. New York: Teachers College Press, 1961.
Kalisch, B. J., & Kalisch, P. A. *Politics of nursing*. Philadelphia: Lippincott, 1982.
Knowles, M. S. *The modern practice of adult education*. New York: Association Press, 1970.
Lorig, K. An overview of needs assessment tools for continuing education. *Nurse Educator*, 1977, 2(2), 12–16.
Malfetti, J. L. Selecting the content of a health education course on the basis of the needs of students. *Research Quarterly*, 1955, 26, 163–169.
Monett, M. L. The concept of educational need: An analysis of selected literature. *Adult Education*, 1977, 27, 116–127.
Stevens, B. J. Nursing leadership: Survival and promise. In S. Ketefian (Ed.), *Perspectives on nursing leadership*. New York: Teachers College Press, 1981.
Survey shows a million RNs employed. *American Nurse*, 1980, 12(9), 1; 6; 10.

Response

Keville C. Frederickson

The dissemination of knowledge and how to apply it is the role of educators. Following formalized education, this task becomes the responsibility of continuing education and the continuing educator. The study utilized ideas and theories from several disciplines to analyze the continuing education needs of nursing's leader elite.

O'Connor (1982) has identified two broad areas generated by the incidents—managerial and human relations; however, the response focuses on two specific categories: communication skills, in providing information in a rational manner; and performance evaluation. These two categories represented almost 43 percent of all reported incidents. Also of interest is that nurses reported twice as many ineffective incidents with performance evaluation as effective. When the emotional overtones of anger are added to these two problem areas, the implications for power and its use in politics becomes very apparent.

Ineffective communication, difficulties with evaluating performance, and anger in nurse leaders inhibits action and is at the heart of political problems faced by nursing and women today. It is these behaviors and feelings that diminish group effectiveness and achievement of goals. Evaluation is a prerequisite for change and the ability to communicate needs and differences, first to each other as a step toward unification and then to legislators and the general public for political influence and policy making. It is the pervasiveness of anger that complicates the situation. A lack of knowledge of cognitive deficits are more easily corrected through continuing education than are emotional or affective problems. One way of viewing these problems is through a psychological-developmental framework.

Developmentally, nursing has not yet arrived at a stage where nurse leaders can use political strategies consistently. By viewing anger and communication problems as developmental in the evaluation of nursing, the outlook is more promising and provides direction. Using a framework such as ego psychology, the early phases of dependency include childlike naivete in which the child depends on the environment to care for him. In fact, the environment is falsely perceived as being all-knowing and protective (Loevinger, 1976). This fantasy allows submission, dependency, and, in the case of nursing's beginnings, political unawareness and inactivity. The physician and/or hospital will acquiesce to the "take-care-of-me" attitude. Also, in this phase of development there is an insensitivity to differences. The view is that everyone is alike.

The next phases of ego development include differentiation, greater autonomy through the awareness that independence is possible; and self-criticism which leads to anger which is present during this phase (Loevinger, 1976). The anger is also generated by the frustration and awareness that we have been duped. The environment is not all-caring and in our best interests. To improve the situation, nurses need to care for themselves and the reality of it sinks in. In terms of change, anger often acts as a stimulus for action. This occurs when nurses strike for better wages and/or working conditions. This phase is also reminiscent of the phrase in the film *Network*, "We're mad as hell and we're not going to take it anymore." However, to move forward into the final phases of adult reality, nurses need to put the anger aside. Gardner (1961) talks about decision-making criteria and the pursuit of excellence. He states that nurses must be aware and accepting of their heritage, the results of historical events and decisions, and their present status in order to project ways in which nurses can reward individual performance (that might be different from current standards) but attain a high degree of excellence. It is this type of attitude that will generate effective political action.

Currently, nurse leaders lack sufficient role models who reflect the adult, reality, ego phase and can provide satisfying interaction. This results in frustration and anger for their staff. O'Connor (1982) found that interactions with nurse superiors (the role models) were most likely to be perceived as ineffective. Therefore, as nurses move up the administrative ladder, they are likely to emulate behaviors learned from nurse superiors. It seems that nurses are teaching and learning ineffective patterns of communication and goal achievement behaviors. Montag used the saying, "Teachers teach as they were taught and not as they were taught to teach." Likewise, it is true that leaders will lead as they were led and not as they were taught to lead.

In O'Connor's study, it is important to examine not only the substance of the findings but also the design. Admittedly, one of the most distressing factors about the study is the exceedingly low response rate. Particularly with this study, such an extraordinarily low return rate poses additional problems. The title indicates leader elite. Elite, by definition, is the "best or most powerful of anything considered collectively especially of a group or class of persons" (The Random House Dictionary, 1980). In considering leadership, a definition that uses graduate education as a criteria is valid. However, leadership elite, by definition, should be limited to a much more select group, for example, members of the Academy of Nursing or Vances' (1977) method for identifying influentials using the reputational method. Another concern is the composition of the respondents since a sampling error is possible. Who has been tested? Given the complexity and time necessary to respond to a critical incident questionnaire, are we considering results that are more linked to nurse leaders and their level of compliance? Are the results more reflective of nurses whose behaviors are based on social desirability, that is, do they do what they think is expected of them or are they the compulsives who use paper as an escape? On the other hand, this population could be the 10 percent of our nurse leaders who are truly professional. Unfortunately, it is not possible to tell or make a judgment on this matter. With a larger group these discriminations might have been made.

Another problem specific to the use of the critical incident method is the sample size. The literature suggests a minimum of 2,000 incidents (Verhonick & Seaman, 1978). It is possible, with such a number in this study relative to what is suggested, that the results may represent the educational needs of one select subgroup of nurse leaders. The critical incident methodology is a difficult one to implement and analyze. Because the sample size required is so large and it is so time-consuming and expensive to implement, few researchers use it. In fact, Verhonick and Seaman (1978) call it a demanding process. However, the information generated by this method is quite unique and valuable when answering questions such as the one raised here by O'Connor. Finding samples and research subjects is becoming a more difficult task. One framework that offers some help with the problem of questionnaire returns is marketing. Many of the skills for successful programming in continuing education utilize a business and marketing approach. Researchers, when colllecting data, are often marketing their questionnaires. Essentially, nurses are trying to sell the subject on the study; asking participants to "buy" the questionnaire. Using marketing techniques, the answers to a number of questions can improve the return on research questionnaires since problems with sampling can invalidate a superb design and consequently the results of the research.

The following are a few ideas:

1. *Is the timing right?* Marketing research had found that brochures or products released during the months of January, February, September, October, and November produce a response rate 30 percent above the average. Those sent during the summer result in a response rate of 10 to 25 percent (Newsletter, 1981).
2. *What is the relationship between the marketing survey (needs analysis) or, in this case, the research and the product we're planning to offer?* Or can we provide what the survey discloses and will anyone buy it if we do provide it?

The leadership group of nursing clearly has continuing education needs. The problem is the size of this group as a market for continuing education. Nurses with a graduate education comprise approximately 8 percent of the total nursing population (American Nurses' Association, 1981). When this group is further limited to those employed in selected educational and practice settings, the group becomes even smaller. Pragmatically, it is not financially feasible to offer continuing education to only this group. More and more continuing education is required to operate as financially self-supporting programs. This group is often too small to provide enough participants and income to be close to a self-supporting program. Also, the usual marketing and advertising techniques of a continuing education unit are usually designed for a general nursing audience within a 50 to 75 mile radius. In order to make such a program successful, a more specialized audience marketing strategy must be initiated. This requires such things as new mailing lists and new advertising approaches. These are expensive, and require more time than many have.

What does work? Nurse leaders with graduate degrees *do* attend workshops; however, they tend to select them based on their need for specific job-related skills. For example, a recent workshop on marketing strategies and continuing education for nurses enrolled almost 60 participants of which almost two-thirds had graduate degrees. The reason for attending they list most often (86 percent) was to improve their knowledge and skills for job-related activities.

The issue that seems to be surfacing here is the connection between identified job-related insufficiencies and topics nurses consider "gaps in learning" that they are motivated to reduce through continuing education. Does the nurse leader presented with a critical incident questionnaire to identify situational inadequacies see its relevance to identified and felt learning needs? In psychotherapy, the answer to this question helps to identify "therapy readiness"; that is, the difference between the patient who acknowledges that a problem exists versus the patient who expresses a willingness to take measures to give up a problem and/or change. Learning readiness as the motivation to change ideas and behaviors is similar. However, returning to psychology, recognition of the problem is the first, and certainly a necessary, step in the process.

The final marketing strategy is follow-up; second and third mailings or reminders are crucial. These always improve participation whether in the purchase of a product, sign-up for a workshop, or return of a questionnaire. In fact, often follow-up mailing will minimize earlier mistakes made with timing of the initial mailing. Experience has shown that the largest percentage of responses usually come from the first mailing but with two well-timed additional mailings the results can equal or surpass the response rate from the first mailing.

In summary—since Dr. O'Connor has stimulated thinking and posed perplexing questions for nurses to consider—it is only fair to elucidate these:

- Since 60 percent of her samples were employed in clinical settings, why were there so few situations related to patient care?
- As leaders in an occupation that focuses on patient care, what is the responsibility for the knowledge base of nursing care?

- Do leaders in similar positions in other patient care-oriented occupations perceive more of their needs as care- or interaction-based?
- What is the relationship between the delivery of nursing care, patient advocacy, and power?

REFERENCES

American Nurses' Association. *Facts about nursing 80–81.* New York: American Journal of Nursing Company, 1981.

Gardner, J. *Excellence: Can we be equal and excellent too?* New York: Harper and Row, 1961.

Loevinger, J. *Ego development.* San Francisco: Jossey-Bass, 1976.

Newsletter. P.S. Market be wise, 1981, 1(4), 3.

O'Connor, A. *Continuing education needs of nursing's leader elite.* Paper presented at nineteenth annual Stewart research conference, New York, Teachers College, April 1982.

The Random House Dictionary, (concise edition). New York: Random House, 1980.

Vance, C. *A group profile of contemporary influentials in American nursing.* Unpublished doctoral dissertation, Teachers College, Columbia University, 1977.

Verhonick, P., & Seaman, C. *Research methods for undergraduate students in nursing.* New York: Appleton-Century-Crofts, 1978.

[8]

The Academic Power of Nursing Deans

Marion D. Lewis

INTRODUCTION

The nursing deanship is acknowledged to be one of the most crucial leadership positions in the profession. It is one in which effects of the incumbent's role enactment extend far beyond the personal rewards and satisfaction of the job. The contemporary nursing dean's potential scope of authority and influence lies both within and outside of the profession in a time frame which may be critical to the future of health care delivery and to the nursing profession. The status and development of nursing, the quality of preparation of nursing practitioners, and the indoctrination of emerging nursing leaders are among the role expectations of educational administrators. Nursing deans are further expected to help establish a secure and equitable place for nursing in national health care planning, to intervene in legislation affecting health care education, and to be assertive spokespersons on issues affecting the welfare of the society.

Such a highly visible and responsible position requires manifold skill and carries a burden of responsibility beyond that which may be borne by the dean's non-nursing counterparts in the university. However, deans of nursing are not only subjected to the universal constraints and pressures of the deanship; additionally, they occupy a unique position in the academic community in that they are primarily women in an historically male environment to which they come from a predominantly female—and historically powerless—profession.

During the last decade there has been increasing concern over the number of nursing deanship vacancies throughout the country. One cause is an apparent lack of willingness on the part of nurses to assume deanships. Various explanations have been postulated to explain why credentialed nurse educators have eschewed the leadership role. Halsey (1978) claims that nurses' negative attitudes toward power militate against their recruitment and retention in administrative positions. Poulin (1975), in the same vein, observes that discussions of power and authority cause anxiety and discomfort among some nurses. Some writers refer to the need to avoid the stress engendered by conflicting role expectations as a plausible explanation of the defection of former deans. Leininger (1974, p. 28) specifically attributes the "Dean's Crisis" to the status, role, and self-image of nurses whose, "socialization fosters attitudes and behaviors dysfunctional to behavior strategies needed for leadership in contemporary times."

A positive outcome of the deanship shortage has been the focus of attention placed on the appropriate preparation of nurses for the still evolving nursing deanship. Anticipatory socialization for aspiring deans and supplementary socialization for incumbent deans is needed. An important component of planned role-learning is a way to assume and exercise the power requisite to fulfilling the dual obligations of university administrator and nursing leader. In writing of the state of nursing in academe, Group and Roberts (1974, pp. 369, 370) state that, "nurses have been abysmally ignorant about the informal power manipulations within universities" and again, "The women who become administrators in schools of nursing are likely to be pawns of the men in power, exercising limited, if any, power of their own." There is a considerable amount of power vested in the nursing deanship deriving from more than one source. The deanship itself is a social identity which carries express grants of power and esteem in the academic world. Further, the nursing dean has ascribed power which accrues from her or his knowledge and leadership position within the profession. It is incumbent on the nursing dean to find ways of energizing power holdings so that multiple role expectations can be fulfilled with competence.

THE PURPOSE

In order to identify the dimensions of socialization that assure successful enactment of the decanal role, further knowledge is needed about those nurses who have already achieved distinction in the role. Since the early 1950s, studies have been done on nursing deans. Most of these investigations were concerned with the nature of their role preparation or with parameters of their role function. No prior study is known which has addressed the relationship between processes of socialization experienced prior to assumption of the decanal role, and the demands of that role. The effects of earlier socialization on dean's perceptions of their role-power is a topic worthy of inquiry as the individual's perceptions define the "real world" in which the role is enacted. Exploration of the relationship between selected socialization factors and present role perception may prove to have significance for planning the professional socialization of future deans. The specific aspects of socialization considered in this study are age, education, and role preparation. All of these might be expected to influence the nursing dean's perceptions of the situation and to directly or indirectly impinge on decanal role-power.

Unlike the socialization factors of education and role preparation which directly impact on role performance, age is an indirect influence which may greatly effect perceptions of self and role expectations. The chronological age of a nursing dean is a general index of the kind of early socialization the person probably underwent in a changing society and the particular values, role norms, and self-concepts internalized. From the age of a dean one might infer the kind of professional socialization into nursing the individual was exposed to in his/her initial educational program (Jacox, 1978).

Nurse training and nurse-roles predominant in the first half of this century served to reinforce and strengthen the sex-oriented socialization of women in our society (Kjervik & Martinson, 1981). Consequently, products of programs of this period could be expected to have greater problems expressing their potential in traditionally male areas of endeavor—for example, the university. Socially imposed barriers to the enactment of power-bearing leadership roles by women and nurses are still existent but are not as imposing or as insurmountable as they once were.

Those nurses whose personal and professional socialization occurred during the post-World War II era would, by comparison, have learned qualitatively different sex-role behaviors and role expectations. Investigation of the relationship between the selected socialization factor of age and the dean's perception of power may support the premise that younger deans hold less restrictive views of themselves in relation to the environment and are less inhibited in their execution of an authority role. On the other hand, findings may suggest that the nurses occupying positions in academic administration are those who have been successful in overcoming the effects of traditional socialization into the nursing role.

REVIEW OF THE LITERATURE

Similarities in the socialization of women and the socialization of nurses in this society have been consistently emphasized in the literature. At any point in nursing history, the status of nursing has been reflected in the status of women; both have been expressions of prevailing sex-role norms. Until recently, nursing has been equated with mothering in that both roles were considered primarily nurturant. Women in both categories have been similarly stereotyped as passive, compassionate, selfless, and dependent; in essence, powerless. In a discussion of the effects of the women's liberation movement on nursing, Group and Roberts (1974) state unequivocally that hospital-based nursing programs are one of the most deleterious elements in nursing. They found that the institutional bureaucracy of hospitals perpetuate the male-dominant, female-submissive social pattern which has typified working relationships between nurses and physicians, and nurses and male hospital administrators. The damage of previous patterns of professional socialization lies in the imposition of a negative self-image which requires the use of subterfuge in order to impart one's knowledge and the masking of supposedly "masculine" traits of initiative and rationality. There is sufficient empirical evidence to support the thesis that many nurses have internalized the nurse-role stereotype which is an extension of their earlier sex-role socialization.

Keller (1979) relates sex-stereotyping to the retarded development of nursing theory. She cites the absence of research emphasis in nursing education and nursing's slowness to develop its theoretical foundations as consequences of nurses' tendency to downgrade their intellectual ability. Many forces serve to perpetuate the impaired self-confidence of nurses, but most perilous of these are the kinds of professional values and occupational identity nurses come to introject during their basic nursing programs. How successful nursing faculty can be in helping to develop positive professional identities in students depends on how successful faculty are in abandoning fallacious stereotypes imposed during their own professional socialization.

Collegiate nursing education may not yet be free of traditional attitudes about nursing, but it represents a giant leap from the guiding philosophy of hospital programs in which the majority of today's nursing deans obtained their basic training. Ashley (1977) helps us to comprehend the psychological effects of repressive socialization by describing the educational patterns of programs which essentially controlled the preparation of nurses in the first half of this century. Apart from being overworked and underpaid (if paid at all), students contracted to observe obedience, respect authority, and demonstrate absolute loyalty on threat of dismissal. Nursing education was, in fact, an apprenticeship whereby learning was achieved by observing, imitating, and performing skills. Through the exploitation of nursing students and denial of their educational and human needs, the hospital-based programs contributed significantly to the devaluation of nursing and its practitioners. The most pervasive disservice was the inculcation of feelings of inferiority and subordination which many nurses carried over into their later careers.

The incongruity between the traditional professional socialization of nurses and the expectations placed on nurses to exhibit attributes of professionalism was addressed by Jacox (1978). A major criterion of a profession is autonomy, accruing from the specialized knowledge and social commitment of its members. "Professionals" are thereby recognized as competent to control the practices and practice settings of their field. However, this notion is in direct opposition to the high value that nursing has traditionally placed on obedience. Jacox observes that faculty in collegiate schools of nursing are still struggling to acquire the autonomy over educational policy and personnel matters in their units that is practiced by their colleagues in other units. One may speculate that nursing leaders have not escaped the limiting role concepts, learned directly and indirectly through professional socialization, which are dysfunctional to effective execution of a leadership role. Sarbin (1968) defines self-role congruence as the degree to which qualities of the self—traits, values, or beliefs—and requirements of the role exhibit fittingness or overlap. His studies led him to the conclusion that "incongruence between self and role creates a state of tension and cognitive strain, which may be the mediating factor leading to less efficient performance" (p. 525). This concept has relevance for nursing deans for whom administrative role expectations are contradictory to the values and behaviors that were expected of nurses at the time they entered the profession. It may be surmised that problems of self-role congruence account for the abdication of some former deans from the administrative position. Of greater interest is the number of nursing deans who have managed to subdue or bypass earlier socialization, through the force of personality or countersocializing experiences, in order to fulfill a role of power and authority with competence and confidence.

CONCEPTUAL FRAMEWORK AND VARIABLES OF THE STUDY

The variable, age, was treated as an historical socializing factor which was included in the study in order to learn whether it has any relationship to the deans' perception of power. In the conceptual framework of the study, three historical periods are taken as having relatively different effects on the socialization processes of the members of the society. Accordingly, it is expected that deans who were born in 1945 or later will perceive themselves as being relatively high in role power; deans born during the 1930 to 1945 time period may have somewhat greater difficulty perceiving their role power as high; and deans born prior to 1930 might be expected to have the greatest problem in viewing themselves as powerful.

The variable, education, applies to role learning acquired in an academic, degree-granting institution. It was anticipated that those deans with a high level of academic preparation for the role would perceive themselves as having a high degree of role power.

The variable, role-preparation, was used to describe extracurricular programs of learning specific to the decanal role, as well as learning acquired through academic or administrative positions held prior to the current deanship. Those respondents who had had specific role preparation were expected also to view themselves as being high in role power.

It was assumed from the literature on role theory that those nursing deans who perceive themselves as holding a high degree of role power will be those who rank high in total role learning. Role theory also proposes that an individual's perceptions of the situation in which a role is enacted influence the effectiveness of role performance. A dean's perception of her situation within the university is revealed by how she perceives her own and her counterparts' role power. Actual power and enactment of power are proposed to be functions of the dean's perceptions of power.

PROBLEM STATEMENTS, ASSUMPTIONS, AND DEFINITIONS

This study was concerned with three research questions. They were:

1. How do deans of nursing perceive their power in functional areas of the decanal role?
2. How do deans of nursing perceive the amount of power they hold as compared to the amount of power their counterparts hold?
3. What relationship exists between the selected factors of socialization (age, education, and role preparation) and perceptions of decanal role power?

The assumptions of the investigator were that:

1. The deans of nursing under study met the same criteria for ap-

pointment to an academic deanship as did their counterparts in the employing institutions.

2. Within universities, all heads of professional education programs who have the title "Dean" are on the same level of hierarchy within the organizational structure.

3. The socialization variables under study impact upon power and perceptions of power in the decanal role.

A relevant limitation to the study relates to the fact that academic administrators of collegiate nursing programs who bear titles of "Dean," "Chairman," "Head," "Director," and so on, share common role-sets and are frequently described by the generic "dean." In order to delineate a particular role as it is found in the organizational structure of most universities, and so that unambiguous counterpart comparisons might be facilitated, the study was limited to those nurse administrators who bear the formal title "Dean." The "counterparts" with whom they were compared are chief academic officers of other professional education programs who have the title "Dean," are employed in the same institution, and function in the same capacity as the dean of nursing.

The operational definition of "power," as used in the study is this: The ability of an academic dean to influence the course of events within the educational unit and the university, through the exercise of implied role prerogatives, authority, and personal leadership skills.*

METHODOLOGY

The survey method was the approach selected for this exploratory study. A two-part questionnaire was mailed to 112 female nursing deans who met the following criteria:

1. An earned doctorate.
2. Administrator of a nursing education unit accredited by the National League for Nursing Council of Baccalaureate and Higher Degree Programs.
3. Assigned the formal title "Dean" by the employing institution.
4. Employed in a university which has one or more other professional education units headed by administrators with the title "Dean."

---

*Six functional areas were used as indices for measurement of power: university affairs, budget, faculty, students, curriculum, and professional affairs.

Part I of the instrument consisted of nine items. Five of these elicited data on the dimensions of socialization under study—age, education, and role preparation. Two items were included to provide information about the dean's tenure in her present position, and the number of counterparts with whom she could make comparisons. The last two items invited the respondent to indicate the categories of individuals she considered influential to her career decision, and the kind of role preparation she found to be most significant to her role performance.

Part II of the instrument included 24 items, equally distributed among six areas of role-function specific to the academic deanship: university affairs, budget, faculty, students, curriculum, and professional affairs. For each function the participant was asked to respond on two identical five-point scales from which her own and counterparts' powers were influenced.

In its entirety the questionnaire was less than three printed pages in length. It could be completed within 10 minutes. The covering letter explained the general purpose of the study and its expected significance. It further encouraged subjects to add comments if they wished, assured confidentiality, and promised an abstract of the report upon completion of the study.

Members of the population were initially identified from the official list of the National League of Nursing Council of Baccalaureate and Higher Degree programs which gives the names, titles, and school addresses for chief academic officers of all accredited programs. From this source, 125 administrators were found who had the academic title "Dr.," the functional title "Dean," and were in a university setting. Verification of status of individuals and their institutions was achieved by cross-checking three other published documents.

The 112 deans invited to participate represented public, private, and sectarian universities in 43 states. In terms of formal education, 58 hold the Ed.D., 49 hold the Ph.D., and the remaining five have other doctorates—Dr. P.H., D.N.S., Sc.D. The nursing deans comprising the sample attended 48 different universities for doctoral study. However, 30 percent of all degrees were awarded by only two institutions: Teachers College, Columbia University (24 degrees), and New York University (9 degrees).

The size and geographic dispersion of the population necessitated use of the questionnaire for data collection. The format of the instrument used adequately provided data relevant to the research questions. Two areas of data were considered essential to the study: (1) the socialization factors under study—age, education, and role preparation; and (2) perceptions of deans' and counterparts' power in decanal role functions.

Selection of items in Part I was directed by the research questions and the selected socialization variables. Categories of role function in Part II were validated through an exploration of the literature which described the major responsibilities of academic deans. Specific items for each of the six categories were compiled from research-generated information. The items were further validated and refined through the pilot study, and consultation with experts in the field of academic administration.

A three-page questionnaire, with covering letter and self-addressed envelope, was mailed to 112 nursing deans. Correspondence was addressed to each dean by name, at her school. Five weeks after the first mailing a follow-up letter was sent to those who had not yet responded. In it, deans were asked to indicate any obstacle to their participation at the bottom of the letter. Subsequently, a second questionnaire was sent to deans who reported having lost or misplaced the original. Eighty-eight usable questionnaires, representing 78.5 percent of the target population, comprise the body of data which were subjected to analysis.

FINDINGS

On the basis of the data provided by 88 respondents, certain conclusions have been drawn about deans of nursing in American universities. They have been summarized and are presented in the order of the research questions.

1. Deans of nursing as a group perceive themselves as having a high degree of role-power in the functional areas which are related to university affairs, budget, faculty, students, curriculum, and professional affairs.

2. Deans of nursing perceive their overall role-power as equivalent to the overall role-power of their counterparts. In the functional areas related to faculty and curriculum, deans of nursing perceive themselves as having a significantly higher degree of role-power than do their counterparts.

3. There is no significant relationship between any of the socialization factors (age, education, and role preparation) and the perceptions of power held by deans of nursing.

It is not possible to devise a profile of deans of nursing in regard to their educational or experiential preparation for the decanal role; these aspects of socialization are too widely varied. There are only two descriptive conclusions that may be drawn from this study: (1) Respondent deans are equally distributed into two age groups—35 to 50 years and over-50 years. (2) Incumbent deans of nursing are similar in the way they perceive power and remarkably dissimilar in those personal experiences which were expected to impact upon perceptions of power.

SUMMARY AND RECOMMENDATIONS

The conceptual framework of the study was based on a belief that certain factors of predecanal socialization would influence the way nursing deans perceive power, and that perceptions of role-power would reflect role performance. The findings revealed a lack of any consistent pattern among deans regarding the socialization factors of age, education, and specific role preparations. Although one investigation is not a sound basis for any definitive statement about these relationships, there is an indication that the processes of socialization studied have no meaningful significance to how deans will perform in the role.

The sample represented over 75 percent of the total population of university-based deans of nursing who are women with doctoral preparation. Most of the respondents are well-known within the profession and have achieved distinction as educational and administrative leaders. Yet it was found that there were great inconsistencies in the scope and content of their role preparations. Of further interest is that 57 of the 88 had received their basic nursing education between 1930 and 1950, a period when professional socialization of nurses was considered repressive of the behaviors needed for leadership roles. From these findings one can only speculate that there are other factors of socialization which have supremacy over the particular socialization processes considered in this study.

Sarbin (1968) had indicated that the learning conditions of early life are important for the acquisition of personal characteristics which result in effective role enactments in later life. He viewed aptitude for a role as the main source of role skill which is only *improved* (but not attained) through appropriate instruction and practice. This theory is supported by Merton (1969): "The styles of leadership . . . are, to an unknown degree, an expansion of the personality structure and early socialization of the leader" (p. 2616). The implication derived is that nursing deans have inherent aptitudes for leadership. Evidence from this study contributes to the implication. An overwhelming number of deans consider their "Personal Qualities and Abilities" *most* significant to their role achievements. Further, it may be inferred that the personal qualities which are conducive to effective role performance in the deanship are transmittable between different kinds of leadership positions. One notes that Hall et al. (1981) found that a major route to the deanship was through leadership roles in professional organizations.

It is apparent that an important aspect of socialization for the decanal role are experiences which enable the prospective dean to recognize, acquire, and exercise power. Such learning would be facilitative to one occupying a potentially powerful role in academe. There is an implicit relationship between qualities of leadership and the ability to use—and to perceive—one's role power.

Conceptual associations of power, leadership, and personality characteristics are found repeatedly in the literature. For example, Urwick (1943) stated that the power of administrative leaders is a function of their knowledge, skill, and personal qualities. Nursing deans themselves have recognized the interlocking relationship of power, leadership, and personal abilities (Christman, 1977; McNally, 1979). The nature of the special characteristics which comprise leadership potential, and the specific nature of early socialization experience which instill these characteristics, is still imperfectly defined.

An implication drawn from the findings of this study is that leadership aptitudes, inculcated through early life experiences, permit the individual to utilize and synthesize previous learnings and to use them in the enactment of a specific role. This assumption would explain inconsistencies between deans' preparations for the role (as inferred from perceptions of power).

The variable age, which was used in this study as an index of the sex-role and nurse-role socialization a dean was likely to have experienced, cannot be completely discounted as an influence on later role behavior. However, the findings indicate that a fuller investigation of early socialization processes is needed. Professional socialization, as such, may well prove to be a negligible factor in the formulation of leadership aptitude since personal characteristics and behavior modes have been established by the time a student first enters nursing. The nursing program then becomes one of many possible settings in which beginning nurses practice and refine their already possessed personal skills. The findings of this study may provide a point of departure for further studies on the nature, source, and development of aptitudes which personify deans and other nursing leaders.

If one assumes that nurses who take on the leadership role of an academic deanship are those who possess personal leadership abilities, some plausible explanation is sought for the respondents of this study who perceived themselves as having a low degree of role-power. It is of significance that the deans of nursing who ranked low in their power to execute various decanal role functions also perceived their counterparts as having low degrees of role power. These findings suggest that role performance within a given institution is dependent on the organizational structure and administrative philosophy of the institution. It is likely that nursing deans, as well as other academic deans, employed by universities in which the degree and scope of nominal power granted role incumbents is severely restricted, will experience role ambiguity and eventual role dissatisfaction. One speculates that the setting rather than the role may have been responsible for the resignations of some past nursing deans.

IMPLICATIONS FOR THE PREPARATION OF NURSING DEANS

Strategies of professional socialization for the nursing deanship can develop but cannot create leadership skills predictive of success in the role. Preparation strategies, therefore, must follow identification of individuals who exhibit personal characteristics and abilities consonant with academic leadership. Frequently the process of self-selection will bring candidates to the foreground; they are likely to have formulated career goals and planned their own progression toward the deanship.

Doctoral study is a basic educational preparation for educational leadership but there is adequate evidence that the major concentration of doctoral study will have little or no significance to future effectiveness in the decanal role. Content in management theory, finance, and organizational structure can provide baseline understandings facilitative to deanship functions. However, the talents and personal skills deans themselves have claimed to be important indicate that educational preparation in communication and interpersonal competence would equally contribute to effective role performance.

Wilson (1972) has said that the tendency to minimize the importance of professional leadership in higher education has resulted in haphazard methods of developing administrative talent. He favors methods of systematic indoctrination such as apprenticeships for prospective academic administrators. One may argue that many nursing deans fulfill their role expectations satisfactorily without benefit of anticipatory socialization. However, the findings of this study related to specific role preparation activities must be looked at very closely. Although no significant relationship was found between continuing education and role-power, more of the deans who had high levels of continuing education perceived themselves as having higher degrees of role-power than did those who had no continuing education preparation. This finding suggests that an orientation to the specific leadership functions of the nursing deanship—through seminars, workshops, or mentor relationships with role incumbents—would contribute to the self-confidence of role aspirants and provide opportunities for "informal political learning experiences" it behooves deans to know (Fagin & Maraldo, 1981, p. 26).

A similar implication is found for another aspect of role preparation. While it was concluded that perception of power is not related to duration of administrative experience, 65 respondents claimed that "Experiential Preparation for the Role" was significant to their achievements in the deanship. On these grounds, it may be recommended that aspiring deans avail themselves of intermediate leadership positions in which they might practice and enhance their aptitudes for management, decision making, and communication.

IMPLICATIONS FOR THE SELECTION OF NURSING DEANS

As a result of her study, Jones (1977) concluded that conceptual and human skills are more important than technical skills for academic administration. Of the deans who met criteria for inclusion in this study, fewer than 20 percent had received their doctorates in educational administration. In view of the scope of educational and experiential backgrounds found among presently functioning and assertively effective nursing deans, it would appear that the curriculum vitae may be the least valid evidence on which to base the selection of a dean of nursing. Deans are recruited from the entire pool of doctorally-prepared nurses. The academic credential implies that the holder has acquired competencies in scholarship, critical thinking, and methods of inquiry, regardless of the major course of study. It is important then to identify those candidates who possess personal qualities and characteristics which promise effective leadership of the educational unit, its faculty, and students. The task of search committees is made easier when applicants for a deanship have established reputations of administrative competency through other positions in higher education. However, if leadership ability is a demonstration of innate qualities developed throughout one's life experiences, assessment of a candidate's performance in other professional roles should be equally predictive of his/her performance in the deanship. Certainly desired personal qualities, as reported by the deans (humor, patience, tact, vision, sensitivity) can be detected during the series of interviews that have been institutionalized into the selection processes practiced in American universities.

REFERENCES

Ashley, J. *Hospitals, paternalism and the role of the nurse.* New York: Teachers College Press, 1977.

Christman, L. Decision making in the academic environment: A dean's viewpoint. In *National League for Nursing, Decision making within the academic environment.* New York: Author, 1977.

Fagin, C. M., & Maraldo, P. Health policy in the nursing curriculum: Why it's needed. *Nursing and Health Care,* January 1981, *30,* 24–27.

Group, T. M., & Roberts, J. I. Exorcising the ghosts of the Crimea. *Nursing Outlook,* 1974, *22*(6), 368–372.

Hall, B., Mitsunga, B., & de Tornyay, R. Deans of nursing: Changing socialization patterns. *Nursing Outlook,* 1981, 92–96.

Halsey, S. The queen bee syndrome: One solution to role conflict for nurse managers. In M. E. Hardy & M. E. Conway, *Role theory: Perspectives for health professionals.* New York: Appleton-Century-Crofts, 1978.

Jacox, A. Professional socialization of nurses. *The Journal of New York State Nurses Association,* November 1978, 6–15.

Jones, P. S. Identification of competencies essential to effective administration of baccalaureate nursing programs (Doctoral Dissertation, George Peabody College for Teachers, 1977). Dissertation Abstracts International, 1977, *38,* 245a.

Keller, M. C. The effect of sexual stereotyping on the development of nursing theory. *American Journal of Nursing,* September 1979, *79*(9), 1534–1586.

Kjervik, D. K., & Martinson, I. M. *Women in stress: A nursing perspective.* New York: Appleton-Century-Crofts, 1981.

Leininger, M. The leadership crisis in nursing: A critical problem and challenge. *Journal of Nursing Administration,* 1974, *4,* 28–34.

McNally, J. The deans' role in baccalaureate and higher degree colleges of nursing. *NLN News,* September 1979, 3.

Merton, R. K. The social nature of leadership. *American Journal of Nursing,* December 1969, *69*(12), 2614–2618.

Poulin, M. A. The nurse administrator: Survival in the executive jungle. *The Journal of the New York State Nurses Association,* December 1975, 9–15.

Sarbin, T. R. Role theory. In G. Lindzey & E. Aronson, *The handbook of social psychology* (Vol. 1). Reading, Massachusetts: Addison-Wesley Publishing Company, 1968.

Urwick, L. *The elements of administration.* New York: Harper & Brothers, 1943.

Wilson, L. The leadership function. In *Shaping American higher education* Washington, D.C.: American Council on Education, 1972.

Response

Erline P. McGriff

Dr. Lewis has provided an operational definition of "power." She has also identified six functional areas used as indices for measurement of power. Her operational definition of power focuses on the parameters of the educational units and the universities. This definition, therefore, is restrictive since the role prerogatives of deans in any setting today must extend beyond university walls and into other social and political systems in the world at large.

The relevance of the study becomes obvious when one reviews the related literature and indeed observes the "deaning" scene in nursing today. A report just published by the American Association of Colleges of Nursing illustrated the length of time in which 240 nursing deans had been in their present positions in 1981–1982. This report represented 240 chief administrative officers in baccalaureate and higher degree programs in nursing. The term "dean" in the AACN study was used in the generic sense with reference to the chief administrative officer of the educational unit in nursing regardless of local title. Fifty-four percent had served for three or less years. The median period of time for the group as a whole was three years as compared to four years in 1980–1981. This percentage must take into consideration, however, that deans of new schools were included in these numbers (AACN, 1982).

Many synonyms and other words have been used for the term "power" and its meaning. They include authority, influence, obedience, control, dominion, prestige, jurisdiction, and command. These, in turn, have been used in describing political and social sway.

One clearly sees a relationship of these concepts to the political arena. For example, how does power relate to politics—a science dealing with the regulation and control of people living in society, influencing policies, and governing activities concerned with achieving advancement or some other group goal, with group pressure and pressure groups? What policies, then, are formulated? By whom? For whom? What course of action is selected from among alternatives to guide, determine, and perhaps control present and future decisions?

One sees that most organizations and particularly colleges and universities are political systems. The concept of power and its distribution and use in contemporary society are concerns of many individuals and groups today in community power structures as well as in complex organizations.

The survey method seemed appropriate for this exploratory study and for the gathering of the data being sought. However, the fact that the sample included only those deans "assigned the formal title, 'Dean' by the employing institution" places a significant limitation on this study.

It would be interesting to see a comparative study done with educational administrators of nursing units in universities who have not been assigned the formal title "Dean" and who may not have a high degree of role-power in the six functional areas studied, particularly the budget.

It might also be revealing to relate the perceptions of power to the specific functional areas of budget. For, in the aspects of organizational politics, the interaction of the internal life with the external environment is paramount. The power of money is a well-known and documented fact (Bretton, 1980).

This respondent noted with pride that the two institutions awarding 30 percent of all degrees to deans invited to participate in the study were Teachers College, Columbia University and New York University. However, the fact that there has never been an autonomous school of nursing with a dean of nursing in either institution must be noted.

I would have liked to have seen more inclusion and treatment of the unique position of the nursing deanship in the academic community, that is, as Lewis indicated, "women in an historically male environment to which they come from a predominantly female—and historically powerless—profession."

Janeway described power as a process of human interaction that takes place between interacting members of a relationship, for example, the powerful and weak, the rulers and ruled, the governor and governed. She continued to state that women are the oldest, largest, and most controlled group of human creatures in the wide category of the weak and the ruled. It was then pointed out that women have some advantages, namely: freshness of vision; lives full of lessons in flexibility; and a deep awareness of life itself as a process (Janeway, 1980).

It has been pointed out that once women started "seeping into the male establishment in large numbers, they brought with them, as their dowry, their own way of doing things, based on their own feelings and views." Woman power is both an additive and catalyst. And, woman power must not underestimate its own strength (Kellen, 1972).

The author agrees with Lewis' finding that "role performance within a given institution is dependent upon the organizational and administrative philosophy of the institution" and hastens to reiterate a finding in her own doctoral research and later from her empirical experience and observations that administrators (deans) in nursing must work cooperatively with others in the university because no one program functions in a vacuum. However, unless the school of nursing has the wholehearted support of the university administration, it is unrealistic to expect that the goals of the nursing program will be achieved (McGriff, 1967). Therefore, the author also concurs with Lewis' finding that the "setting rather than the role may have been responsible for the resignation of some past nursing deans."

The author is distressed with the implications for the preparation of nursing deans that "there is adequate evidence that the major concentration of doctoral study will have little or no significance to future effectiveness in the decanal role." This finding that specific role preparations seemed to indicate that they might not be meaningfully significant as to how deans will perform in the role was intriguing. In the author's own doctoral research, the investigator concluded that there was a need for a specific role preparation for educational administrators in nursing. Therefore, the author believes that administrators of nursing programs need knowledge, understanding, and skill in three major areas: nursing, administration, and higher education (McGriff, 1967). In knowledge there is power but more possession of knowledge is not enough. It must be augmented by control over the application of this knowledge.

In the First Annual Helen Nahm Research Lecture, Meleis (1981) pointed out that "in its search for professional identity and meaning, nursing has proceeded through several ages," namely, the age of practice, education, and administration, research, nursing theory, and scholarliness. If now is the time for the age of nursing scholarliness, then nursing must liberate itself from its parochial trappings and use its scholarship accordingly in education, administration, and research.

Nurses, and particularly educational administrators, must hold themselves in high esteem and refrain from all tendencies to "downgrade their intellectual ability, impair their self-confidence" or any other qualities that jeopardize our professional values and identity.

The author is not at all certain that the position dean of nursing requires "manifold skill and carries a burden of responsibility beyond that which may be borne by the dean's non-nursing counterparts in the university." This aspect was not studied in the report by Lewis, and the author believes nursing education administrators must use caution in making such generalizations about nursing's being different. It is the author's opinion that non-nursing counterparts also have "dual obligations" and the responsibility to fulfill "multiple role expectations with competence." The author believes that responsibilities for deans in institutions of higher education are essentially the same regardless of the nature of the educational program being administered.

Two other questions might be raised here with regard to further explorations in this general area. How do the nursing deans' counterparts perceive their power-status and how is the power of deans perceived by the central administration and indeed by the faculty?

Cohen (1980) writes that "all power is based on perception. If you think you've got it, then you've got it. If you think you don't have it, even if you have it, then you don't have it" (p. 12).

I summarize with a quote by Janeway:

> Inventing the future—metaphorically—drafting a map that will fit it—is an active process of learning and collaboration. . . . The past was full of surprises; the present is astonishing; who knows what the future may be . . . let us not lay out a planned and structured utopia, but work toward a map of uncertain prediction connecting to memory, a map of promise, a map of possibility, of an unbounded future that will not be limited by an end. (Janeway, 1980, p. 9)

REFERENCES

American Association of Colleges of Nursing (AACN). *Report on salaries of nursing deans in colleges and universities.* Washington, D.C. 1982.

Bretton, H. L. *The power of money.* Albany: University of New York Press, 1980.

Cohen, H. *You can negotiate anything.* Secaucus, N.J.: Lyle Stuart, Inc., 1980.

Janeway, E. Powers of the weak (1st ed.). New York: Knopf, 1980.

Kellen, K. *The coming of age of woman power.* New York: P. H. Wyden, 1972.

McGriff, E. P. *Administrators of graduate programs in nursing as educational leaders.* Unpublished doctoral dissertation, Teachers College, Columbia University, 1967.

Meleis, A. I. *The age of nursing scholarliness: Now is the time.* The First Annual Helen Nahm Research Lecture, June 19, 1981. San Francisco: School of Nursing, University of California.

9

Public Policy Making on a Nursing Issue

Patricia Ruth Mixon

INTRODUCTION

In an effort to examine systematically how public policy is determined on a nursing issue at the state level of government, a field study was conducted which explored the policy making process in the state of Florida on an issue that impacted directly on nursing practice.

An interview schedule, designed to prove the policy process, was the primary instrument utilized to collect data for the study. It was utilized with key participants on the issues. Additional research data were obtained from organizations' minutes, personal files of participants, government documents and proceedings, newspaper articles, and the investigator's observations of the committee deliberations when the nursing issue was considered by the Florida Legislature during its 1978 legislative session.

FLORIDA'S NURSE PRACTICE ACT PROPOSED AMENDMENT

On April 28, 1978, a bill was introduced in the Florida Senate that, if passed, would have substantially revised the Nurse Practice Act. Senator Jack Gordon, a Democrat from Miami Beach in his second term of office, sponsored the bill and was responsible for initiating it. Senator Gordon was known to be antiphysician in his district and in the Florida legislature. He had served as chairman of the Senate Health and Rehabilitative Services Committee (HRS) and was currently vice chairman of the Senate Appropriations Committee, Chairman of the Finance,

Taxation, and Claims Committee, and a member of the HRS Committee.

Senator Gordon had sponsored legislation at past sessions related to cost containment and he was a strong advocate of measures that would control the spiraling cost of health care services in all areas of the health care delivery system in Florida. Many bills that Senator Gordon had sponsored in connection with the health care delivery system had been actively opposed by organized medicine.

It was clear to Senator Gordon, who had looked at a variety of ways to save the state money in his former position as chairman of the Senate HRS Committee and in his more recent position as vice chairman of Senate Appropriations, that a nurse practitioner could provide certain medical services to needy persons and that by purchasing these services in lieu of physician services, the state would save money. Senator Gordon's motivation on this issue was his goal of controlling the spiraling cost of health care services in the state of Florida. He felt that health care costs had to be contained prior to the institution of any new programmatic scheme for national health care services.

The first provision of Senate Bill 1038 (SB) amended the definition of the practice of professional nursing by deleting a provision that permitted an advisory committee composed of members of the Board of Nursing and the Board of Medical Examiners to decide what additional acts are proper to be performed by nurses licensed under Chapter 464.021 (4), Florida statutes (FS). The first provision authorized the Board of Nursing to decide by their own rule what constitutes specialized and advanced levels of nursing practice in the nursing profession.

A second provision specified that the rendering of nursing services on a fee-for-service basis, or the reimbursement for such services, or the establishment of an independent nursing practice are not prohibited by law. This would allow for third party reimbursement for nursing care and could encourage nurses to establish private nursing practices.

A third provision required by the Department of Health and Rehabilitative Services (DHRS) to provide to eligible recipients of medical assistance the services of an advanced registered nurse practitioner (ARNP) who was certified under Chapter 464. FS. In addition to the federally required Medicaid services, the DHRS would make available to eligible recipients the services of a certified ARNP in accordance with Title XIX of the Social Security Act.

The DHRS estimated that SB 1038 would save money for the publicly funded Medicaid Program, since nurse practitioners would be reimbursed at a lower rate than would physicians. It also estimated that any increase in utilization resulting from eased access to medical services would be offset by reduced cost to the individual client. The DHRS reasoned that utilization of nurse practitioners in underserviced areas would tend to ease access for all recipients in need of medical services.

Gordon introduced SB 1038 in the Senate; afterwards it was referred to the Senate HRS Committee for a hearing on May 15, 1978. The committee adopted a technical amendment by Senator Gordon at the request of the Florida Nurses Association (FNA) which deleted language that defined nursing services as acts within the scope of the nursing license or when appropriate physician input had been received.

After public testimony by Ms. Mary Finnin, RN, representing the FNA and all categories of ARNPs, and by Mr. Scotty Fraser, representing the Florida Medical Association (FMA), the bill failed to pass on a 3 to 3 tie vote. A motion was made by Senator Jon Thomas, chairman of the Senate HRS Committee, to reconsider the vote by which the bill failed as a courtesy to Senator Gordon, but the bill was not brought up for reconsideration the following week. On May 22, 1978, by rule of the Senate, the bill was reported unfavorably.

When the nursing bill was not brought up for reconsideration in the Senate HRS Committee, Ms. Marcia Beach, legislative aide for the Broward County delegation and spokesperson for Senator Jon Thomas, suggested that the concept was premature for the Florida legislature to deal with at this particular time and that the votes were not there to reconsider the bill. Ms. Beach suggested that possibly the introduction of the issue by Senator Gordon was only the first step on a long-range political strategy to legislate one of many measures to support health care cost containment in Florida. Another interpretation of the failure to reconsider the nursing issue is that debate among the committee members might have put legislators who were up for reelection in the fall in the posture of antimedicine or antinursing.

BACKGROUND SURROUNDING THE ISSUE

The first licensure law regulating the practice of nursing in Florida was enacted in 1919, and in 1975 the act was substantially revised to reflect current concepts of the expanded role of the nurse as a health care provider in the health delivery system. The strongest move for statutory recognition of an advanced level of practice which the revisions incorporated originated in south Florida. The Board of Nursing was authorized at the time of the revisions to adopt rules concerning the authority of various categories of nurse practitioners to perform particular acts and it was authorized to certify nurse practitioners in specialized categories.

When the Nurse Practice Act was revised in 1975, inclusion of the term "diagnosis" as a function in the statutory definition of nursing practice resulted in intense interaction between organized nursing and organized medicine, which strongly opposed the use of a term that traditionally had been reserved for the practice of medicine being applied to nursing functions. As a compromise, an amendment which had originated with the FMA was adopted by the legislature which created the advisory committee with the stipulation that the advisory committee be composed of three members from each board for nursing and medicine for the purpose of recognizing additional acts to be performed by nurse practitioners.

Conflict between the FMA and the FNA was exacerbated at both the 1976 and 1977 legislative sessions. In 1976, a bill sponsored by Representative Hodes which failed to be heard in committee would have mandated a one-year internship for nurses seeking a Florida nursing license. (Representative Hodes was a physician.) At the 1977 session, a bill that provided for geriatric outpatient clinics under state supervision and funding to be staffed by registered nurses was successfully amended at the request of the FMA to include the utilization of physician assistants in these clinics to provide patient services.

Events following the creation of the joint advisory committee suggest that the committee was unable to achieve the purpose for which it had been created. After two years of faulty meetings between representatives of the two boards, a consensus of agreement on what constitutes additional acts to be performed by the nurse practitioners could not be reached. Finally, in 1977, the Board of Nursing took the initiative and promulgated rules and regulations pertaining to the functions of nurse practitioners without approval of the designated members who represented the Board of Medical Examiners.

In implementing the revisions of the act, the Board of Nursing determined categories of Advanced Registered Nurse Practitioners to include: (1) Certified Registered Nurse Anesthetist; (2) Certified Registered Nurse Midwife; (3) Geriatric Nurse Practitioner; (4) Family Nurse Practitioner; (5) Pediatric Nurse Practitioner; (6) Adult Nurse Practitioner; (7) Clinical Nurse Specialist (i.e., cardiovascular, obstetric, orthopedic, pediatric, respiratory, and psychiatric-mental health); (8) School Health or College Health Nurse Practitioner; and (9) Adult Primary Care Nurse Practitioner. The ARNPs were organized in 1977 as a section of the FNA and assumed executive responsibility as a member of the Board of Directors.

In the spring of 1978, the Board of Nursing began certifying its first ARNPs in the various categories for advanced levels of practice after concluding that ratification of a list of additional acts by physician members of the advisory committee would not be forthcoming. The Board of Nursing felt that its decision was based on firm ground since the committee had received considerable input from both physicians and nurses practicing in the various clinical specialties. Additionally, the Board of Nursing interpreted the law to mean that it had the final authority to promulgate the rules and regulations for an advanced level of nursing practice. The Board of Nursing considered nurses who were certified under other certifying agencies, such as the American Association of Nurse Anesthetists and the American College of Nurse Midwives, as being eligible for certification.

Concurrently, as the Board of Nursing was preparing to certify its first ARNPs in the spring of 1978, the Board of Medical Examiners advised the Board of Nursing that medical members of the joint advisory committee could no longer meet with nursing members for this purpose until a ruling was made by the attorney general on what constitutes proper additional acts to be performed by the ARNPs.

In the meantime, the FNA's Board of Directors voted to oppose the proposed Appendix B of the rules and regulations for the ARNPs which listed, as additional acts, acts that were currently being done by registered nurses within the scope of the nursing license. The FNA requested that the Board of Nursing consider only prescription of medications and performance of minor surgical procedures as being in the category of additional acts since all other functions that were listed in the rules and regulations were already within the nature and scope of nursing practice. Action by the Board of Nursing on the recommendations that were proposed by the FNA's board of directors on the Appendix B was temporarily passed until the next advisory meeting of the Board of Nursing on May 15, 1978.

Related to the nursing issue is the fact that, in 1977, the FNA won a statewide election to act as the collective bargaining agent for approximately 3,000 health care professionals employed by the state. The bargaining unit is comprised of registered nurses, physicians, dentists, pharmacists, nutritionists, occupational therapists, physician assistants, psychologists, and speech therapists. Subsequently, Ms. Finnin, RN, representing the FNA, acted as bargaining agent for a nurse who had been fired by the state. The case involved staffing patterns of public institutions which permitted unlicensed individuals to administer medications to patients rather than nurses licensed by the Board of Nursing.

During this period, both the FNA and the Board of Nursing had repeatedly taken the position that administration of medications is a nursing function and should not be performed by individuals who were not licensed by the Board of Nursing. In connection with the staffing patterns of public institutions that permitted and provided for the administration of medications by aides, the FNA had requested the Board of Nursing to exercise its authority under Chapter 464. FS to prevent programs authorized by the DHRS to train aides in the administration of medications for public institutions.

In connection with the nursing issue were the activities of Ms. Terri Brower, RN, project director of the Geriatric Nurse Practitioner Program at the University of Miami. Ms. Brower, RN, had been involved in a personal research project during this period which focused on the nurse practitioner movement and legislative change. Ms. Brower, RN, had written and spoken to various legislators about the need for statutory recognition of the ARNPs who were experiencing severe obstacles to full utilization of their skills in the employment field. A limiting factor on nurse practitioners entering into joint practice with physicians was attributed to reluctance of physicians to sign reimbursement claims for services performed by the nurse practitioner rather than the physician.

Ms. Brower, RN, was also a member of the Nursing Home Ombudsman Committee (NHOC), and had been instrumental in getting the recommendations of the committee to members of the House and Senate HRS committees. The NHOC, whose purpose was to receive, investigate, and resolve complaints against nursing homes in Florida, had been created by state statute in 1975. The NHOC had recommended as one of its priorities that ARNPs be recognized by the DHRS as providers of health care services in both inpatient and outpatient health care facilities in the private and public sectors.

Compounding the nursing issue was the issue of a separate department of health in Florida. Since 1975, when the department of HRS was last reorganized and relocated in Tallahassee, many attempts had been made by organized medicine to separate medical matters from the total structure of DHRS and create a separate department of health. Organized nursing supported the concept of a separate department of health and thus became allied with organized medicine. Senator Gordon strongly opposed attempts to create a separate department of health and thus gave organized medicine bureaucratic control over the health care system in Florida.

INTEREST GROUP ACTIVITY

Prior to the time that the nursing issue surfaced at the legislative session, neither organized medicine nor organized nursing was aware of the provisions of the bill, although the FNA had been contacted by a senate analyst and by Senator Gordon's administrative aide about the issue. Senator Gordon made the decision to pursue legislation that would lessen physician control over nursing practice without direction from either of the two groups most affected by the issue. Immediately after initiating the nursing issue and a few weeks prior to the time the session was convened, Senator Gordon directed Mr. Abrams to solicit the American Association of Retired Persons (AARP) and the state Association of Condominium Owners for support on the issue. Senator Gordon was a member of the State Health Coordinating Agency, as was a representative of the AARP who provided him with direct information on the problems of senior citizens in obtaining health care services on fixed incomes. Senator Gordon had attended meetings for purposes of identifying and resolving problems associated with health care of the elderly, and he was aware of the concerns of the AARP.

The AARP, which has over 950,000 members in Florida, supported the bill since it would have increased the accessibility of preliminary health care services provided by the nurse practitioners to the elderly more economically than services provided by a physician for the same services. However, the AARP did not lobby the bill after it was introduced at the session.

When the nursing issue surfaced at the session, it quickly activated the FNA and the FMA, the two groups that the issue most directly affected. Since the bill was filed late in the session, neither organization had much time to develop and implement lobbying activities. Within a week after the bill was introduced in the Senate, it was scheduled to be heard in the Senate HRS Committee. However, it was deferred to the following week due to a crowded Committee agenda.

The FMA maintains four fulltime lobbyists in Tallahassee who routinely monitor the development of legislative proposals throughout the year. The FNA, on the other hand, has either one or two individuals who routinely lobby for the organization. Their base of operation is the FNA's headquarters in Orlando, except during legislative sessions when the lobbyist resides in Tallahassee.

The FMA was not opposed to the concept of the nurse practitioner as long as the nurse practitioner's functions were performed under the immediate supervision of a physician. However, the FMA opposed the issue on the grounds that nurse practitioners' fees were to be paid out of an already limited amount funded by the DHRS for physician services.

It was the opinion of the FMA that the advisory committee, mandated by the 1975 statutory revision of the Nurse Practice Act, should not be disbanded since the committee performed a valuable function in the interests of qualifying acts for the ARNPS. According to the FMA, independence of the Board of Nursing in promulgating the rules and regulations of the ARNPs could be construed by the courts as negating and violating current concepts of the Medical Practice Act in Florida.

The chairman of the FMA's Allied Health Committee cited possibilities of physician exploitation of nurse practitioners in independent practice as a factor related to the position of the FMA on the nursing issue. In the chairman's opinion, it was not a question of nurses functioning in an expanded role, which the FMA supported, but one of physician control of those functions that were being performed by a nurse practitioner. Physician supervision had to be in operation at a level that was congruent with the reality of the situation. This could not be achieved when a physician set up X numbers of ARNPs in practice for X amounts of dollars a day and made rounds on the practitioners once or twice a day, and in the process made "little slaves" of the ARNPs. Thus, it was the opinion of FMA that a mechanism of control for this type of exploitation had to be built into any legislation concerning the practice of the ARNPs.

After the nursing issue surfaced at the legislative session, Mr. Scotty Fraser, representing the FMA, was immediately in touch with the president of the FMA and the chairman of the Legislative Council for directions on how to lobby the issue. The issue was reported by Mr. Fraser to the FMA's House of Delegates which was in session at the time. Following this activity, Mr. Fraser alerted the FMA's constituents at the local level to be in touch with their respective legislators, especially the members of the Senate HRS Committee, to voice the FMA's opposition to the issue and to get the bill killed in committee.

Mr. Fraser and one other lobbyist for the FMA contacted each member of the Senate HRS Committee individually, with the exception of Senator Gordon, to voice the FMA's opposition to the issue. Mr. Fraser and his associates used a list of specific functions that had been promulgated by the Board of Nursing to point out specifically to committe members "just how far nursing had gone." Additionally, the FMA's lobbyists concentrated their lobbying efforts on two members who were considered to be uncommitted or swing votes—Senators Childers and Vogt.

The FNA supported the concepts in the bill. Ms. Finnin, RN, representing the FNA, testified before the Senate HRS Committee on May 15, 1978 that the association strongly supported direct reimbursement of Medicaid funds and third-party payments for nursing services. The 1978 legislative plank of the FNA supported legislation which provided for third-party payment for nursing services.

The FNA supported the provision that specifically deleted the Advisory Committee to the Board of Nursing on the grounds that the physician members consistently presented delay tactics, even to the point of boycotting meetings, which had the effect of obstructing the promulgation of rules and regulations of the ARNPs. Additionally, the

FNA opposed the Advisory Committee on the grounds that there was not a similar statutory provision that provided for nursing input to the Board of Medical Examiners on medical acts. The FNA supported the provision that addressed the right of independent practice, although it was the opinion of the FNA that nurses could currently practice on a fee-for-service basis on their current nursing license. Above all else, the FNA was strongly opposed to economic suppression of nursing by organized medicine which, according to Ms. Finnin, RN, constitutes antitrust activity: when one profession attempts to control another profession and reap economic benefits from that control.

When the issue surfaced at the session, Ms. Finnin, RN, expressed the FNA's position on the issue to members (or their staff) of the Senate HRS Committee. Ms. Finnin, RN, also alerted and requested support on the issue from the Florida Board of Nursing and from various nurse leaders around the state, then published the information on the issue in *The Florida Nurse*. Ms. Finnin, RN, asked several nurses to be in touch with their respective legislators to support the issue. Ms. Finnin, RN, also contacted the Public Health Nursing Program Supervisor, Ms. Dolores Wennlund, DHRS, for support of the FNA's position on the issue.

In an analysis of the bill, Ms. Wennlund noted that local health units could expect that health care services would be more accessible and economically delivered which could lead to an increase in demand for health care services. Ms. Wennlund pointed out that it was timely and appropriate to recognize the independent role of nursing in the provision of health care, however, the joint advisory committee should be retained to address problems ensuing from the overlapping functions of medicine and nursing. Ms. Wennlund, who routinely analyzes bills of this kind that have an effect on the levels and amount of public health care services, also pointed out that some heat would be generated at the local level as a result of organized medicine's resistance to the issue. While Ms. Wennlund may initiate a certain amount of support or opposition for a health or nursing issue by alerting the nursing supervisors in local county health departments and nursing consultants within the DHRS, she did not do it on this issue.

After the nursing issue was heard in the Senate HRS committee on May 15, Ms. Finnin, RN, unsuccessfully attempted to arrange a compromise with the Senate HRS staff and Senator Gordon's administrative aide to delete the language of the first two provisions of the bill, leaving the provision that addressed reimbursement by third-party payment intact since this was a priority of the association.

Senator Jack Gordon prefiled the nursing issue in November 1978, SB 1, for consideration of the 1979 Florida Legislature. A newspaper article in the *Florida Times-Union* (December 2, 1978) noted that the nursing issue is aimed at broadening the scope of the Advanced Registered Nurse Practitioners. The article quoted Senator Gordon as saying, "The whole thrust of the issue is to make use of the personnel available" and "The real issue is—can a nurse practice without a doctor's say-so?" (*Florida Times Union*, p. B1). Senator Gordon called the proposed legislation a cost containment measure which is part of a package of bills that he planned to introduce at the 1979 legislative session to cut the cost of health care in Florida.

KEY PARTICIPANTS

Many activities of participants in the policy process on an issue are overt and expected, and clearly link individuals to issues. It is obvious that certain individuals who are identified in the making of public policy, such as the governor, the legislature, private and public interest groups, and the press participate in the making of public policy. But which individuals and groups were key participants on this issue, which was narrow in scope and which primarily affected nurses?

First, there was no evidence that the press played a role in the policy process on this issue. The press, generally, is concerned with broader issues that affect large numbers of individuals and issues that generate a high level of controversy in all phases of the deliberative process. This issue did not fit these criteria.

Next, individuals who played key roles in the policy process on the issue were not always easily identified by other participants. For example, while all the participants on the nursing issue knew that Senator Gordon sponsored the issue, only Mr. Abrams was aware that Senator Gordon initiated it. Activities that occur in connection with one issue do so in competition with many other issues which often have priority status for the individuals who are involved in the political process. These kinds of background conditions contribute to unclear links between activities and individuals in the policy process.

Key participants on the issue were representatives of the state associations of organized medicine and nursing which had been in existence for many years and were well organized to develop and monitor legislative proposals at the Capitol and to lobby issues that concerned the organizations. The involvement of organized medicine and nursing on the issue was expected because, generally, legislation that affects nursing will interest medicine.

While the role of the FNA is to be quite active in monitoring and lobbying bills during the legislative session which concerns them, it is organized medicine which exercises power and shapes legislation that affects the scope of nursing practice in Florida.

Other organizations, such as Florida National Organization of Women (NOW) and the AARP, have the potential for effectively shaping policy issues that directly affect nurses, but they did not exercise this power. These groups lacked political experience, had a scarcity of resources, and had other priorities.

None of the organizations which were involved on the issue were political organizations or had a political ideology. Political parties were viewed by the participants as not playing a significant role on the issues. Generally, party or party affiliation was not viewed as a channel of access to the policy process.

There was no evidence that either the Florida Board of Medical Examiners or the Florida Board of Nursing were directly involved or played key roles on the issue. Generally, board members do not concern themselves with issues that do not affect the parameters of safe nursing practice. The nursing issue was evaluated by the Board of Nursing as not being critical to the functioning of the board and did not warrant more attention than the activities that were provided by Ms. Finnin, RN, of the FNA, according to the executive director of the Florida Board of Nursing, Ms. Helen Pat Keefe, RN.

The Florida Board of Nursing and other professional and occupational regulatory boards in Florida had been advised by the legislature not to testify before a committee on an issue unless specifically called to do so by the legislature and not to engage in lobbying activities unless legislation directly affects the functioning of a board. While lobbying activities are not specifically prohibited by the legislature, the general intent was to prevent regulatory boards, advisory committees, and other agencies of the state of Florida from lobbying an issue with a strong self-interest motivation. The directive of the Florida legislature to the Board of Nursing and the DHRS was congruent with trends and philosophies in other states regarding the concept that regulatory agencies of government become self-sustaining over time. This had the effect of limiting the role that the Board of Nursing played as an overt participant on the nursing issue.

HOW POLICY DECISIONS WERE INFLUENCED

One of the most difficult aspects in analyzing how decisions on policy issues are made is to determine how, when, and by whom influence is exercised in relation to a policy decision. A general explanation, however, can be sought by objectively looking at the strategies and tactics utilized by individuals and groups to influence events on an issue.

The events and activities in connection with the nursing issue, SB 1038, have to be viewed in terms of the overall political strategy of Senator Gordon, sponsor of the bill, who had a reputation of high credibility. While the influence of the powerful FMA was apparent on this issue's short history, it was quite obvious that the introduction of the nursing issue in this legislative session was only the first step in a long-range political strategy of Senator Gordon's to lessen the control of the nursing profession by organized medicine in order that the state could eventually purchase services of ARNPs in lieu of physicians' services whenever this arrangement was feasible.

The fact that the bill did not get out of committee was not relevant in Senator Gordon's long-range political scheme. It was Senator Gordon's style to introduce a bill primarily for the purpose of bringing an issue before the public and to the attention of the legislature for debate either one or two legislative sessions in advance. For as as long as health care cost containment measures remained a priority with Senator Gordon, the bill would be reintroduced at succeeding sessions by him until legislation in some form was passed by the legislature.

Senator Gordon's immediate goal was to involve two stable organizations of elderly and condominium owner citizens on the issue in order to later establish a link between these individuals, many of them beneficiaries of the Medicaid program, and the services of the ARNPs. This strategy had the effect of broadening the interested public which is important from a political standpoint.

At the legislative session, Senator Gordon used the nursing bill as a red herring to divert the attention of both the FMA and the FNA from other issues, especially the issue creating a separate department of health. Senator Gordon hoped to break up an alliance that existed between the FMA and the FNA both of whom advocated a separate department of health in the state. Senator Gordon was strongly opposed to creating a separate department of health out of the DHRS on the grounds that it was illogical to separate out specific health measures from other measures that contribute to health and, in the process, give physicians immense control over health matters in the state bureaucracy.

Nursing, in the meantime, was unwilling to have the Nurse Practice Act opened up for revisions in fear that undesirable changes would be legislated once Chapter 464 FS was before the legislature. Since third-party payment was a legislative priority of the FNA for the session and was addressed as one of the provisions in the nursing issue, the FNA's attitude that the Act would undergo undesirable revisions when it was before the legislature was clearly inconsistent with their priority to address this problem.

The committee hearing on the nursing issue, which gave the appearance of little controversy and without real interest to either organized medicine or organized nursing, was misleading, considering the relevance and significance of the issue to both professional groups. None of the provisions was debated adequately and the impression was that the 3 to 3 tie vote on the issue in the Senate HRS Committee on May 15, 1978 was a matter of the votes being settled prior to the hearing and the other two positive votes reflecting respect for Senator Gordon by Senators Vogt and Childers.

The position of both the FMA and the FNA remained unchanged throughout the period and neither organization was willing to compromise on the basic issue of who was to control nursing practice. The FMA was committed to maintaining medical supervision over nursing acts, and nursing was equally adamant in its position that the medical profession was extreme in its approach of medical supervision over nursing acts since this was not being done in the field currently. In fact, it had never been done. A further motivating factor that strengthened organized nursing's position on the nursing issue was organized medicine's economic suppression of nursing which the FNA considered clearly illegal.

The activities of Ms. Brower, RN, in connection with her personal research and in relation to her position as project director of the Geriatric Nurse Practitioner Program at the University of Miami, appeared minimal and ineffective. Working alone, Ms. Brower, RN, was able to achieve only slight recognition for her efforts. The recommendation to utilize ARNPs for geriatric patients came out of the State Nursing Home Ombudsman Committee in which Ms. Brower, RN, was involved and may have influenced some legislators.

Ms. Finnin, RN, who represented organized nursing, was well known and had maintained high visibility throughout the political system during the past decade. That Ms. Finnin, RN, was known as the bargaining agent for professional employees in the state and, as such, was considered to represent a union and to wear two hats did not diminish her reputation as chief negotiator for professional nurses in the state.

While Ms. Finnin, RN, testified in support of the nursing issue and requested support of committee members, she did not utilize concrete data relative to the practice of the ARNPs to persuade legislators to vote for the nursing bill in committee. Mr. Fraser utilized a list of descriptive acts that were being performed by nurse practitioners to convince the undecided members of the Senate HRS Committee to oppose the issue. However, there is no clear evidence that Mr. Fraser's activities actually persuaded the three members of the Senate HRS Committee to vote no on the bill when it was heard in this Committee.

The final decision on the nursing issue in the Senate HRS Committee had no meaning in terms of a win or loss for any group since the Committee hearing on the bill was only the first step in a long-range political strategy of the sponsor, Senator Gordon.

RECOMMENDATIONS

Based on the way public policy is made at various levels of government, the research data of this study, and the values of the researcher, the following recommendations are made for professional nurses who are interested in increasing their influence in the political arena of policy making on issues that concern them:

1. That professional nurses be ever alert to subtle changes in society that require statutory recognition and initiate legislative proposals on both professional and health care issues. The issue in this study had its origins outside of nursing; however, state nursing associations are organized by their structure and purposes to protect the interests of nurses in these areas. For greater political effectiveness, professional nurses should organize themselves more completely by joining their state nursing association (members provide wealth and visibility to an organization)* and implement the following strategies:

- Plan well in advance for legislation that the organization is interested in initiating. Long-range planning increases the probability of successful passage through the legislature.
- Secure the services of individuals with political expertise who are familiar with the issue and have expertise in the specific issue area several months before an issue is to be introduced in the legislature to assist in the development and implementation of political strategies to achieve statutory change.

---

*Utilizing data available at the time of this study, it was estimated that only 10 percent of registered nurses licensed by the state to practice were members of the Florida Nurses Association in 1977–1978. However, approximately 89 percent of physicians licensed by the state in the same time period were members of the Florida Medical Association.

- Secure cooperation of other legislators who have positions of power, such as chairmen of key committees, before the legislative session is convened.
- Contact legislators, especially key committee members, before the legislative session is convened to inform the members about the issue. Be brief, concise, and concrete in presenting information to legislators who have neither time nor inclination to deal with lengthy submissions from individuals and groups.
- Develop position papers on legislative issues and goals and disseminate to legislators, paying particular attention to members of key committees where bills that affect nurses are heard. Committees are key decision points in the deliberative process.
- Seek to influence the vote on the noncommitted member of key committees. The data suggested that legislative committees function as a pivot for those members who may vote either way.

2. That professional nurses be prepared to develop and implement political strategies during legislative sessions other than from a defensive, reactionary posture. In this study, Senator Gordon's plan was not fully communicated to organized nursing which placed them in a defensive posture at a critical time during the policy process.

3. That professional nurses can expect opposition on policy issues that deviate from the traditional view of the functions of professional nursing, and be prepared to deal with opposition of organized medicine and other individuals in the polity who support the traditional view of a nurse's functions. Firmly entrenched in our society is the concept that the physician is the primary health care provider, and any policy issue that challenges the right of the medical profession to control all aspects of health care functions will be met with strong resistance by organized medicine.

4. That professional nurses develop political awareness in the making of public policy, which is based on a process of bargaining to gain political objectives. The process of bargaining is continuous as old values and existing laws are constantly challenged from year to year in the political arena. Government staff provide direction and stimulation for much of the bargaining and compromise among individuals and groups.

5. That professional nurses and other proponents of change of policy issues be prepared to overcome obstacles at many different points in the policy process. The political system is a negative system and tends to maintain the status quo of existing law. The complicated bill-passing procedures and the formalized rules of procedure by which state legis-

latures make laws serve as obstacles to change. In addition, custom and traditional ways of thinking and doing resist change and help to maintain status quo.

6. That professional nurses be aware that there are many different access points to the policy making structure and that critical points are choice of sponsors for a bill and key committees.

7. That professional nurses develop and maintain high political visibility in a state by participating in voting and supporting legislative candidates and incumbents who endorse legislative goals of organized nursing.

8. That professional nurses develop and maintain rapport with legislators at the local level by nurse constituents in legislative districts. The research data suggest that legislators listen to their constituents' problems and attempt to resolve problems by either initiating or supporting issues that meet their constituents' needs.

9. That professional nurses develop and maintain open communication with administrative aides, legislative analysts, and other government staff in a state. These individuals occupy important positions in the political system which enable them to function in liaison roles on policy issues. They also have the capacity to control information, an important political resource, on policy issues.

10. That organized nursing maintain its present local, state, and national organizational structure to provide a mechanism for expression of the wishes of the majority of nurses on legislative goals. The structure also provides for input of information, direction, and support from the national level. The research data in this study suggest supporting an organized effort, in lieu of individual effort, to gain political objectives.

11. That professional nurses develop and maintain open communication with like-minded individuals and organizations; that organized nursing overtly support policy issues which originate with these groups and that are congruent with legislative goals of professional nurses. This supporting action will benefit professional nurses by building good will, another important political resource. Many of these individuals and organizations are potential recipients and employers of nursing services and good will contributes to the employability factor.

12. That professional nurses participate in high-level health planning to increase the probability of influencing the development and implementation of public policy on health issues. To gain this objective, professional nurses should seek positions of importance in state government for which they qualify to effectively implement political strategies of organized nursing.

REFERENCES

Florida Times Union. December 2, 1978, p. B1.
Senate Bill 1. Florida Senate, 1979.
Senate Bill 1038. Florida Senate, 1978.

UNSTRUCTURED INTERVIEWS

Abrams, Mr. Dave, Administrative Aide to Senator Gordon (District 35), Miami, Florida, August 1978.
Beach, Ms. Marcia, Spokesperson for Senator Jon Thomas and Administrative Aide to the Broward County delegation (District 30), Coral Springs, Florida, August 1978.
Brower, Ms. Teri Francis, Project Director, Geriatric Nurse Practitioner Program, University of Miami, Miami, Florida, August 1978.
Carroll, Mr. Jack, Volunteer lobbyist, American Association of Retired Persons, Tallahassee, Florida, October 1978.
Finnin, Ms. Mary J., Executive Director, Florida Nurses Association, Orlando, Florida, July 1978.
Fraser, Mr. Scotty, Director of Legislative Affairs, Florida Medical Association, Tallahassee, Florida, July 1978.
Gordon, Senator Jack, Senate (District 35), Tallahassee, Florida, November 1978.
Keefe, Ms. Helen Pat, Executive Director, Florida Board of Nursing, Jacksonville, Florida, August 1978.
McCallister, Mr. Syd, Legislative Analyst, Florida Senate, Tallahassee, Florida, June 1978.
Perez, Dr. Louis, Chairman, Allied Health Committee, Florida Medical Association, Sanford, Florida, August 1978.
Sodec, Ms. Beth, Staff, Nursing Home Ombudsman Committee, Tallahassee, Florida, July 1978.
Wennlund, Ms. Dolores, Health Program Office Supervisor, DHRS, Tallahassee, Florida, July 1978.

SUGGESTED READINGS

Bauer, A., & Gregens, K. J., (Eds.). *The study of policy formation.* New York: Free Press, 1968.
Bauer, R. A., Pool, I., & Dexter, L. A. *American business and public policy.* New York: Atherton Press, 1963.
Blair, G. S. *American legislatures: Structure and process.* New York: Harper and Row, 1967.
Campbell, R. F., & Mazzoni, T. L., Jr. *State policy making for the public schools.* Berkeley, Calif.: McCutchan, 1976.

Clark, T. N., (Ed.). *Community structure and decision making: Comparative analyses.* San Francisco: Chandler, 1968.

Dahl, R. A. *Modern political analyses.* (2nd ed.). Englewood Cliffs, N.J.: Prentice-Hall, 1970.

Dye, T. R. *Politics in states and communities.* (2nd ed.). Englewood Cliffs, N.J.: Prentice-Hall, 1973.

Easton, D. *A systems analysis of political life.* New York: John Wiley and Sons, 1965.

———. *A framework for political analysis.* Englewood Cliffs, N.J.: Prentice-Hall, 1970.

Gross, B. M. *The legislative struggle.* New York: McGraw-Hill, 1953.

Jewell, M. E. *The state legislature.* New York: Random House, 1962.

Key, V. O., Jr. *Politics, parties, and pressure groups.* (5th ed.). New York: Thomas Y. Crowell, 1964.

Lindblom, C. E. *The policy making process.* Englewood Cliffs, N.J.: Prentice-Hall, 1968.

Lockard, D. *The politics of state and local government.* (2nd ed.). New York: Macmillan, 1969.

McConnell, G. *Private power and American democracy.* New York: Alfred A. Knopf, 1966.

Meranto, P. *The politics of federal aid to education in 1965.* Syracuse, N.Y.: Syracuse University Press, 1967.

Schneier, E. V. (Ed.). *Policy making in American government.* New York: Basic Books, 1969.

Truman, D. B. *The governmental process.* New York: Alfred A. Knopf, 1951.

Usdan, M. D. *The political power of education in New York state.* New York: The Institute of Administrative Research, Teachers College, Columbia University, 1963.

Wahlke, J. C., Eulau, H., Buchanan, W., & Ferguson, L. C. *The legislative system.* New York: John Wiley and Sons, 1962.

Wilson, F. A., & Neuhauser, D. *Health services in the United States.* Cambridge, Mass.: Ballinger, 1974.

Zeigler, H., & Baer, M. A. *Lobbying: Interaction and influence in American state legislatures.* Belmont, Calif.: Wadsworth, 1969.

Response

Janet N. Natapoff

A public policy is a course of action selected by government and directed toward some end. Put simply, it is what governments do and do not do. Dr. Mixon's study demonstrates how policy is made and what influence nursing has on the process.

The theme of this book underscores the importance of not only policy, but power and politics as well. Power enables a group to influence others through the political process. The result is policy. Entry into nursing practice, the scope of this practice, and health care financing are all determined by policies at the national, state, and local levels. Despite increasing interest in the use of power, politics, and policy by nursing, few researchers have explored how policy is actually formulated. Dr. Mixon's study focuses on the analysis of policy formulation.

Dye (1972), a political scientist, emphasizes the importance of describing and exploring the causes and consequences of governmental activity as a way of understanding public policy. Dye has described several models which are useful as frameworks for studying policy. Using one of these models, Kalisch and Kalisch (1982) outline several stages in the policy making process, each of which can be identified in Dr. Mixon's study although she did not explicitly outline a framework for analysis.

Dye (1972) states that policy research involves describing and explaining the causes and consequences of governmental activity by outlining the content of policy, analyzing the impact of environmental forces, institutional arrangements, the results of political processes on policy formulation, and, finally, the evaluation of the consequences of the policy on society. Dr. Mixon has taken the first several steps. Further research is needed to complete the process to evaluate the consequences of policy as well as its formulation.

The issues selected for study by Dr. Mixon are important for both health care and nursing. The two she defined as having a direct effect on nursing, the Nurse Practice Act revision and midwife reimbursal, are crucial issues in many states. A review of the "News" section of the *American Journal of Nursing* revealed that the state policy issues were discussed more than 20 times since January of 1981. The vast majority of these news items were concerned with the same two issues Dr. Mixon studied. In New York State, third-party reimbursement for community-based nurses and for nurse midwives is being reviewed in committees. There are also several bills which propose to amend the Nurse Practice Act. Because her issues are still with us, nursing should pay careful attention to her study findings.

Dr. Mixon used an exploratory field study approach to analyse the selected issues, an appropriate methodology for examining relationships as they exist in real life (Polit & Hungler, 1978). Because field studies examine real life processes, data should be obtained from participating actors. She mentions an interview schedule which was utilized with participants but does not give the framework for this schedule. It is not clear how much of her excellent analysis is based on primary sources nor is it clear what instruments were used to collect data.

Assuming her sources are valid, it is disturbing that nurses were not among her list of key participants. Nurses apparently exerted little or no influence on issues which clearly affected their practice, even when that effect could be considered positive. Instead, nursing issues were used by others for their own purposes. The Kalisches (1982) define policy makers as those with authority or legitimate power to allocate resources. The policy-making process has many points of access and interest groups can and do impact on policy decisions. The American Medical Association is a powerful interest group that has been able to influence policy decisions and, indeed, is still actively involved in nursing issues in Florida. The American Nurses Association is becoming more powerful and has been able to influence policy makers at the national level. It has been less successful at the state level, as Dr. Mixon's analysis demonstrates.

One way to increase influence is to form coalitions with other concerned groups. Dr. Mixon points out that the recipients of care provided by Advanced Registered Nurse Practitioners were not activated during the Nurse Practice Act Issue. Why not? Significantly, the March of Dimes, a consumer-oriented group, initiated the midwife issue without the assistance of two important groups of nurse midwives. Did the March of Dimes consider the nurses as powerless and, therefore, not solicit their help? Why did the nurses not join forces with the March of Dimes? The importance of forming coalitions with other groups cannot be underestimated, particularly for a group struggling to gain power and therefore influence. The recipients of care are our natural allies. Building such coalitions will help nurses become policy initiators rather than policy recipients.

In her conclusions, Dr. Mixon emphasizes the importance of persua-

sion and bargaining to the political process. Along with these two behaviors go negotiation and compromise. Her conclusions do seem to
be based on study findings and emphasize the necessity for nursing
to learn and use these important techniques. Leininger (1978) defines
negotiation as "the diverse ways and means of coming to an agreement" so that participants believe they "'all won something' from the
negotiations" (p. 2). When nursing is on the receiving end of policy
formulation, as this study shows, it is hard to feel like a winner.

Bargaining and negotiation take place when each participant is fully
activated by the issue and each has something to give and to receive.
It might be helpful for state Nurses' Associations to draw up a list of
"bargaining chips" which can be used during political negotiations.
Nurses in Maryland were able to get third-party reimbursement for all
nurses after first securing it for one group—the midwives. Nurses active in that campaign stress the importance of negotiation and compromise as a legislative strategy. A bill introduced for one specialty
allowed others to follow later (Griffith, 1982; Goldwater, 1982). Nursing can come from a stronger position when it knows what it must
keep, what it can negotiate away, and what it wants from other interest
groups.

Dr. Mixon outlined a list of recommendations which should be dupli-
cated and presented to all nurses. Her steps to success in the political
arena, however, are not easy to follow without the active support of
nurses behind some organized body, presumably the professional association. To become more influential, nurses will have to become more
sophisticated in their understanding of the political process and more
powerful when they negotiate. Senator Inouye, a strong advocate for
nursing, wonders why it always seems that a physician or an economist
is the primary spokesperson for nursing issues and asks, "Why hasn't
the nursing profession utilized the true extent of their potential power?"
(1982). To utilize this power, nurses need to demonstrate their collective worth.

Dr. Mixon conducted a study in an area where there is little literature.
Like any study there are both weaknesses and strengths. The strengths
of this study clearly outweigh the weaknesses. Public policy research
is difficult, and guidelines have not been established. According to the
policy analysis literature, Dr. Mixon's methodological approach was
sound.

Further research in this area is needed. One approach might be to
study legislative campaigns where nurses have had some success. In
some states, such as Maryland, nurses have been able to achieve desired goals. On the national level, nurses have been successful in securing federal funding for nursing education. Finding out why nurses have

been successful in some areas while losing in others might be a major contribution to the profession.

Dr. Mixon's findings should be shared with all nurses. It is crucial for nurses to work together in the political arena. The Nurse Training Act is under attack by the budget cutters. Sunset laws in at least 35 states require periodic review and legislative action on each Nurse Practice Act. Even in states without sunset laws, the practice acts are constantly being challenged by powerful interest groups. Third-party reimbursement is being debated everywhere. To rephrase a common cliche, the health care pie is getting smaller and nurses must fight for their share.

Finally, nurses must recognize that political power is shifting to the states. It is here that future health care decisions will be made. Bloc grants will be distributed by state health care policy makers. The "new federalism" will shift important welfare programs to the states. Adequate funding is essential for all human services. What influence will nursing have when important health and welfare decisions are made? Can nurses use this power to improve health care for clients?

REFERENCES

Dye, T. R. *Understanding public policy*. Englewood Cliffs, N.J.: Prentice-Hall, 1972.

Inouye, D. J. Foreword in B. Kalisch and P. Kalisch, *Politics of Nursing*. Philadelphia: J. B. Lippincott, 1982.

Goldwater, M. Direct third-party reimbursement for nurses: A legislator's view. *American Journal of Nursing*, 1982, *82*, 411–414.

Griffith, H. M. Direct third-party reimbursement for nurses: Strategies. *American Journal of Nursing*, 1982, *82*, 408–411.

Kalisch, B. J., & Kalisch, P. A. *Politics of nursing*. Philadelphia: J. B. Lippincott, 1982.

Leininger, M. Political nursing: Essential for health service and educational systems of tomorrow. *Nursing Administration Quarterly*, 1978, *2*, 1–16.

Polit, D. F., & Hungler, B. P. *Nursing research: Principles and methods*. Philadelphia: J. B. Lippincott, 1978.

10

Dilemmas in Decision Making

Patricia Westbrook Blagman

INTRODUCTION

In the not too distant past, the nursing profession could be likened to the "lady of the castle" of medieval times who was without rights and authority when the lord and master was in the castle. Wits, feminine wiles, and a little deceit enabled her to manage in the system. Yet, when the lord was away, he gave her such significant powers as coining money and raising an army (Mumford, 1970). Today, the castles are gone, and women's relationships with men have undergone great change. There is today a greater assumption of autonomy, authority, accountability, and power on the part of nurses. One can ponder still, has there been enough assumption of the previous virtues to firmly establish the power of nurses in the health care system?

Fortified with new practice acts, nursing has forged into roles involving greater independence and power. Decision making is a component of this independence. Nurses have always made decisions; however, the scope of their decision-making practice was limited and frequently subjected to the control of others. The formulation of a nursing diagnosis used to be an unacceptable decision-making process. Now it is commonplace, important both in chart audits and quality monitoring tools. Decision making related to diagnosis carries with it the foundation for responsibility, accountability, and the ability to assume more power in the health care delivery system.

As nursing strives for more input into the decision-making process at all levels of health care practice, it should be able to gain and yield power effectively. With increased power, a better understanding of the decision-making process and the various concepts associated with the process is necessary.

PURPOSE

The purpose of this investigation was to describe selected variables which influence patient care decisions made by staff nurses. The variables addressed were: values/utility; risk-taking behaviors; and personality characteristics. In addition, relationships between the subject's level of educational preparation, number of years in practice, and modality of care were studied.

Influences on choice behaviors included: decision maker variables; variables concerning alternatives of a specific decision situation; and situational variables. This study examined both decision maker variables and specific decision situation variables.

DEFINITION OF TERMS

Values

Human behavior is governed in large measure by values, that is, by the attractiveness of alternatives (Becker & McClintock, 1967). The decision-making process in many cases represents a compromise between what the decision maker views as the reality and the supposed shared value system (Billings, 1974). "A real life decision involves some goals or values, some facts about the environment, and some inferences drawn from the values and facts" (Simon, 1959, p. 254). The decision-making process is subjective in that values are constantly changing as an individual thinks of each possibility in the decision (Carney, 1971). Each time a nurse makes a decision, the process starts with explicit values or goals and the task is to decide how to make the best choice among available alternatives (Kassouf, 1970).

Utility

When value is considered in nonmonetary terms, it is called utility. Utilities are therefore subjective values (Kogan & Wallach, 1967). In health care arenas, McIntyre, McDonald, Bailey, and Claus all defined value (utility) in terms of therapeutic effect or contribution to patient welfare (1972).

The concept of utility reflects the many dimensions of values. Money frequently serves as a general measure of value, yet it is inadequate as a measure for certain values such as winning a race, having health, or obtaining education.

The concept of utility can provide a basis for relative assessments between concrete choices (Steinbruner, 1974). In the decision maker's mind, one is then able to compare the worth of the choices in comparable terms by making a utility assignment, as in a preference ordering.

The values an individual holds are an integral part of the decision process. They exert their influences in the selection between alternatives.

Risk-taking Behavior

In any decision situation the outcome of an alternative will be: success, failure, or maintenance of the status quo. When the probability that a successful outcome will occur is known with certainty, there is no dilemma for the decision maker. Yet, rarely is this the case. Lack of certainty about the decision outcome and the prospect that the outcome might be failure or loss give rise to the risky nature of the decision process (Kogan & Wallach, 1967). The risky aspect of decision making is pervasive in daily life.

Many definitions of risk focus on the probability that an outcome will occur and the loss if the outcome does not occur. For example, in deciding which horse in a race to bet on, one considers the probability (odds) of the horse to win and the betting price one might lose. The magnitude of both probabilities and losses enter into the determination of the amount of risk in a given situation.

Patient care decision making by nurses is easily identified with risk taking. Nursing decisions may be evaluated in terms of risk to the nurse, the health care agency, and the client (Bower, 1972). In a decision-making study of baccalaureate nursing students, risk was defined as the degree of probability of patient injury, damage, negative benefit, or degree of patient hazard involved (McIntyre, McDonald, Bailey, & Claus, 1972).

Is there a personal value for risk? Do attitudes of individuals differ substantially? To some persons risk is considered good, exciting, and to others it is a danger to be avoided. What may be risk to one individual is another's insurance against boredom (Kassouf, 1970). However, risk taking in itself is a neutral value (Carney, 1971).

Personality Characteristics

Decision theorists have studied the personality patterns of the individual associated with risk-taking behaviors. Researchers have felt that if they were able to identify a constellation of personality traits correlated with risky decision behavior, they might predict risk taking in decision-making situations (Plax & Rosenfeld, 1976).

Achievement motivation has been the most consistent personality correlate with risky decisions. Studies indicate a strong relationship between high need for achievement and the choosing of medium risk alternatives; and between high fear of failure and more risky or more cautious alternatives (Atkinson, 1957; Harnett & Baker, 1974). For example, when there is a high need achievement, the decision maker cannot risk failing and thus chooses an alternative with a medium risk level. In this case, choosing the cautious alternative would insure success but probably not meet the achievement need. When there is high fear of failure, the decision maker can choose the cautious alternative to insure success, or, the decision maker can choose the more risky alternative, justifying a failure on the grounds it was likely to fail.

Researchers have concluded that it is difficult to clearly define a personality pattern associated with risk in decision making.

SAMPLE DESCRIPTION

This chapter studies the relationship between nurses' specific personality traits, rationality, and risk taking in the decisions they make in the care of immobilized patients. Ninety-eight staff nurses, comprising 97 females and one male, from eight New York metropolitan area hospitals, participated in this study. Their ages ranged from 21 to over 45 years. Fifty-one percent of the nurses were 21 to 25 years.

The educational preparation of the subjects were: 41 diploma, 24 associate degree, 31 baccalaureate degree, and 2 with master degrees. Only two nurses in the sample had been in nursing practice less than six months. Most were experienced nurses, with three to 10 years of practice.

The models of care utilized were: team nursing, primary nursing, and individual daily patient assignments. Seventy-seven nurses practiced in a medical-surgical unit, and 21 worked in specialty units such as neurological, orthopedic, and geriatric services.

METHODOLOGY

The Edwards Personal Preference Schedule was used for personality data collection. Information on values and risk-taking behaviors was obtained by the Kogan-Wallach Choice Dilemma Questionnaire (CDQ). Ten nursing dilemmas were constructed to involve nursing decisions for immobilized patients. Three of these dilemmas had a component which involved a potential risk to the nurse as well as the patient. The nursing dilemmas contain identical criteria to the Kogan-Wallach CDQ. In these choice dilemmas, two alternatives are offered. One alternative was cautious, that is, it has a greater likelihood of success but is of lesser value in comparison to the second alternative which was associated with a greater likelihood of failure but was very valuable if successful.

Immobility of patients was the content focus for the nursing dilemmas. It was chosen because of its prevalence in hospital patients. Most complications from immobility can be prevented by independent nursing actions. The goal for the nurse in each dilemma is prevention of complications from immobility.

A five-point scale was used to measure risk. Value was measured by asking the sample to give a value for the cautious alternative, a value for the risky alternative succeeding, and a value for the risky alternative failing. As a second measure of risk behavior, subjects were asked to identify their choice in the situation.

SUMMARY OF FINDINGS

Values/Utility

The utility scales ranged from high, mid, and low values. Respondents were asked to indicate values for the outcomes of each alternative. The group mean for the values of the cautious alternative was 3.5, indicating a low value for this alternative. The group mean for the risky alternative being successful was 7.2, indicating a high value for this alternative. The group mean for the risky alternative failing was 4.8 or of mid-value. This summary indicates that even if the alternative should fail, it is considered of more value in failure than the cautious alternative in success.

Risk-taking Behaviors

Risk was determined by the mean of the probability preferences (level of confidence) for the risky alternative. A score of five was midpoint in the range between cautious and risky. This meant the subjects were neither cautious nor risky.

Risk was also measured by examining the responses as to whether the subjects in a given situation would actually choose the risky or the cautious alternative. In seven of the 10 nursing dilemmas, 78 subjects projected they would choose the risky over the cautious alternative. For the remaining three dilemmas, the subjects preferred the cautious alternative. The subjects were considered risky on this measurement.

A third method for risk measurement was to project how much more risky a subject might have been in a situation and still have been within the framework of selecting an alternative based on their probability preference and value preference. Fifty percent of the choices could have been more risky on this measurement. This is probably the most insightful risk measurement.

Personality Characteristics

Ten personality variables were measured: achievement, exhibition, autonomy, succorance, dominance, abasement, nurturance, change, deference, and aggression. Nurses in this study scored highest in achievement, nurturance, and change. They scored lowest in aggression along with abasement, dominance, and succorance. Exhibition, deference, and autonomy were midrange.

Relationships

Relationships between risk, personality, and demographic variables were analyzed by chi-square. Educational background made no differences (sig. .01) on riskiness between the 41 diploma, 24 associate degree, and 31 baccalaureate nurses. The length of time in nursing practice made no difference in risk-taking behavior. There were also no differences (sig. .01) on riskiness between the three patient care modes: individual, team, and primary nursing. There were no differences between age groups in risk-taking behavior.

This study on nursing dilemmas indicates a lack of willingness to take risk on the part of nurses. It is also probably not surprising that there were no significant relationships between riskiness and the personality variables, except for nurturance. What is significant, however, is how this study supports other research findings. High need achievement individuals made decisions of moderate riskiness. The achievement score was one of the three highest personality variables.

SUMMARY, RECOMMENDATIONS, AND IMPLICATIONS

Staff nurses in this study were neither cautious nor risky. They could have made more risky decisions based on their values.

Decision making is taught as a process in nursing curriculums. What needs to be incorporated into this process is a more in-depth study of the variables which affect this process. Use of decision trees, simulation games, and computer-assisted decision-making studies can help learners experience the outcomes of their decision making and increase confidence in making quality decisions.

The nursing profession appears to be handicapped by its strength of personality variables which reflect the personal caring aspects such as nurturance, without enough strength in the powerful aspects of the personality, for example, autonomy and assertiveness. Nursing has been able, in the past, to refrain from risky decision making by relinquishing to others such responsibility. If one is not accountable for an action, one cannot be blamed for it. The more powerless one acts and the less influence one exerts, the more open to exploitation one becomes.

There is no inherent value in risk. The goal is not to develop risky individuals but rather to develop individuals who are fully able to participate in the decision-making process and be able to take the risky alternative when it is warranted. The goal of autonomous decision making is achieved through education. The effect of the educational milieu on the undergraduate is paramount in providing the student with the opportunity to achieve this goal.

The traditional pyramid administrative model in nursing has contributed to the dependency of those at the base of it, the staff. When decision making is centralized at the top or near it, nurses at lower levels will become passive, dependent, and unenthusiastic (Gillis, 1982). The more dependent one is, the less power one has.

When the traditional administrative model is loosened and decision making is decentralized, staff nurses have more power in the decision making over conditions of their practice. Having more power in decisions over staffing ratios, standards of care, and staff development will increase job responsibility, personal autonomy, job satisfaction, and personal power.

REFERENCES

Atkinson, A. W. Motivational determinants of risk-taking behavior. *Psychological Review*, 1957, 64, 359–371.

Becker, G. M., & McClintock, C. G. Value: Behavioral decision theory. In P. R. Farnsworth, O. McNemar, & Q. McNemar (Eds.), *Annual review of psychology*. Palo Alto, Calif.: Annual Reviews, Inc., 1967.

Billings, C. R. Understanding meta-decisions: The key to effecting organizational change. *Journal of Educational Data Processing*, 1974, 11, 4–5; 8–64.

Bower, F. L. *The process of planning nursing care*. St. Louis: C. V. Mosby, 1972.

Carney, R. E. *Risk taking behavior*. Springfield, Ill.: Charles C Thomas, 1971.

Gillis, D. A. *Nursing management: A systems approach*. Philadelphia: W. B. Saunders, 1982.

Harnett, J. J., & Baker, R. M. Fear of failure in group risk-taking. *British Journal of Social and Clinical Psychology*, 1974, *13*, 125–129.

Kassouf, S. *Normative decision making.* Englewood Cliffs, N.J.: Prentice-Hall, 1970.

Kogan, N., & Wallach, M. A. Risk taking as a function of the situation, the person, and the group. In *New Directions in Psychology III.* New York: Holt, Rinehart, and Winston, Inc., 1967.

McIntyre, H. M., McDonald, F. I., Bailey, J. T., & Claus, K. K. A simulated clinical nursing test. *Nursing Research*, 1972, *21*(5), 429–435.

Mumford, E. The nurse as participant. *New York State Nurses Association Journal*, 1970, *1*, 16.

Plax, T. G., & Rosenfeld, L. B. Correlates of risky decision making. *Journal of Personality Assessment*, 1976, *40*, 413–418.

Simon, H. A. Theories of decision-making in economics and behavioral science. *The American Economic Review*, 1959, *49*(3), 253–282.

Steinbruner, J. D. *The cybernetic theory of decision.* Princeton, N.J.: Princeton University Press, 1974.

Response

Joan G. O'Leary

The intensity of risk taking in patient care decisions was studied by Dr. Patricia Blagman (1981). Selected variables which influence patient care decisions made by staff nurses were analyzed. Decisions were evaluated in terms of risk to: the nurse, the agency/institution, and the patient.

What is the thread that motivates an individual to take risks? Can a positive environment improve risk-taking behavior? A nursing administrator should allow creativity to flourish by fostering freedom of expression. Repressive measures may result in conformity, and one does not grow or develop.

Blagman (1981) identified that achievement motivation was the most consistent personality correlate with risky decisions. An administrator should be sensitive to the fact that high achievers choose medium risk levels in nursing practice.

Decision making is taught as a process in baccalaureate programs. Possibly the development of quality preceptorships could allow the students to synthesize knowledge gained during the academic years and gain decision-making experience in the clinical arena.

Nursing students should be able to put into practice what they have learned about risk taking. Some nurse educators believe that they have been teaching nursing students to be assertive change agents in the hospital system. Many young graduates may believe this is their role, but they soon learn that changes in the hospital do not come easily. Many young graduates today, upon beginning their first work experience, are confronted with a dilemma. Prepared by teachers who are visionary, the neophyte nurse often possesses some skills and knowledge that are presently unmarketable. Educators do tend to emphasize theoretical experiences. More emphasis needs to be placed in the practice area which requires continuous decision-making abilities.

In a school setting, the student nurse has an opportunity for precision and clinical practice in instructed, selected assignments. Procedures are usually not done until they have been supervised. In the academic world, theory precedes practice. The nursing student is often led to believe that there is only one correct way that things should be done. In "real" clinical practice, this certainly does not exist. The nurse clinician is confronted daily with unexplored, unexplained, and fluctuating situations that had never been confronted during the school experience. This can contribute to a minimizing of risk taking because of fear of failure. It becomes more comfortable to maintain the status quo.

Some hospitals have preceptor programs which have a senior student come to the hospital and work side by side with a primary nurse for a period of time. This may be done three to six months prior to graduation. In this type of program, the student can ask questions informally with time to gather data. Decision making then becomes experiential.

The way in which a new graduate elects to resolve "reality shock" eventually influences not only how he or she interprets the first experience as a nurse, but also how he or she views the entire career in nursing. Frankly, it is a disservice to new graduates to send them into a complex environment such as the hospital, deficient in technical skills. They cannot advance to more complex areas if they are hampered by a competence in the fundamentals of nursing practice.

Something constructive should be done about reality shock. Nursing should focus on merging the needs of education and nursing practice.

This may result in increasing autonomy and an improvement in appropriate risk-taking behaviors for the nurse.

There are two aspects about women to consider in the phenomenon of risk taking. One is how women regard their own roles in job-related success or failures; the other is society's expectations of women.

First, let us consider how women view their own roles in their jobs. It has been said that women often maintain negative self-concepts despite positive work experiences. Women have not been socialized to feel successful even when they are; but interestingly, they do regard failure as a reflection on their self-concept. Put more simply, women do not readily accept credit for success, because they attribute success to an easy task or a lucky break. They do, however, accept personal responsibility for failure. Therefore, in nursing, a predominantly female profession, when one is unable to deliver quality nursing care, the nurse believes that it is her fault and that she has personally failed.

There can be no doubt but that the stress and strains on clinical nurses will increase. Health care has become, and will continue to be, much more technological and complex. Major ethical decisions weigh heavily on every health professional as science provides the means for protecting and maintaining life. A number of years ago the staff nurse's daily assignment consisted of patients in varying stages of recovery and illness. Today, the nurse may be required to care for a group of patients who are acutely ill in a critical condition. The acuity of care within the hospital has increased as the length of stay in the hospital has decreased. The nurse's patient caseload may well consist of patients hovering between life and death states, attached to life-supporting machinery. Within this humming, often noisy environment, the nurse is responsible for helping the patient's family and the patient to adjust to a major health problem.

Hospitals, in the ever-increasing desire to reduce expenses, tend to use an industrial model for cost reduction, by providing auxiliary personnel for non-nursing tasks. This may mean that the nurse can hardly leave a unit for lunch because of the critical needs of her patients. Unlike other health professionals who may also have responsibilities toward patients, the nurse is the one professional who never has the opportunity to get away from the stressful environment.

The functional modality, a system adopted by nursing in some hospitals, is a task-oriented system whereby divisions of labor are viewed apart from patients' needs. It can depersonalize nursing care. For example, one nurse administers medications, another gives treatments, and another changes beds. Quantity, deemphasizing quality, is a negative factor in this model.

Team nursing was the answer to the profession in the 1960s. In this model, several nurses, orderlies, and aides were put under the supervision of one particular nurse called the team leader. This nurse was to provide care to a group of patients, approximately 20 in number. Ideally, the Team Leader was one of the best prepared nurses. She had to know not only the diagnosis and the medications, orders, and tests, on each patient, but also the family problems and their social and ethnic backgrounds. She had to compile a nursing history and help the team formulate a care plan on each patient. She also had to supervise the activities of others, hold nursing care planning conferences, and, many times, give medications and treatments. It was not surprising that the burnout occurred and the actual time spent with patients became secondary to the supervisory functions in the team leader model.

Consider the personal cost to the individual nurse. Unable to accomplish all those tasks, the nurse began to disengage. The nurse can no longer allow herself to continue to really care for patients. Treating people as objects is a symptom of dehumanizing behavior. Examples of other types of dehumanizing behavior are evident to anyone familiar with the hospital setting. Withdrawal is another symptom which may occur. The nurse simply finds an excuse to spend less time with patients.

It is evident that less risk taking occurs when the professional is forced to provide care for too many patients at one time. As the ratio of patients to nurses increases, the result is a higher and higher emotional overload until the nurse just burns out and emotionally disconnects. When staff ratios are lower, the individual staff nurse can give more nursing care to each patient.

In primary nursing some of the potential power of nursing is beginning to be realized. The nurse functions as an independent practitioner by assuming the responsibility for the total nursing care of six to eight patients for the 24-hour period. The primary nursing model is similar to the case method on which nursing was originally practiced. Primary nursing allows autonomous practitioners to have a direct line of access to patients, physicians, and other health practitioners. In primary nursing, nurses are responsible for their own practice decisions. They are accountable to patients, peers, professional organizations, and the courts for their conduct.

Autonomy for nursing means the ability to make decisions with patients. It means mutual access between the patient and the nurse without the supervisor or the director of nursing acting as the gatekeeper. The direct responsibility and authority of the primary nurse is in assessment, diagnosis, planning, implementation, and evaluation of care.

Can the model of primary nursing increase autonomy and assertiveness in risk taking? The nurse should be seen as the patient's assistant, not the physician's assistant. Professionally, the nurse should be responsible to the patient. The primary nurse is the patient's advocate and alleviates anxiety associated with hospitalization and illness. The whole patient, with consideration of his or her lifestyle, family, medical history, occupation, and expectations of the hospitalization, becomes the focus of the nurse's care. The patient is seen as an individual who has had his or her life interrupted by illness. The patient usually looks forward to resuming a normal, healthy life, post hospitalization. Primary nursing represents an approach to patient care that emphasizes health and a sense of wellness. To achieve that goal a nurse has to take risks.

The reliance on slavishly following bureaucratic rules impairs risk-taking behaviors. The emotional stress triggered by the nurse's taking responsibility for unpopular or painful decisions can sometimes be avoided if he or she tells the patient and/or family, "These are the rules and I have to follow them." The author does not wish to imply that health workers should throw caution to the wind and break rules designed to protect patients, institutions, or staff. Some rule books, however, are heavy enough to fall off shelves in nursing stations and hurt somebody! The point is that rules should be subjected to careful interpretive nursing judgment. As Dr. Blagman stated in her study, "Nursing has been made to refrain from risky decision making and if one is not accountable one cannot be blamed."

The nursing administrator should apply understanding and interpretation to all cogs of the wheel in leadership. The values and beliefs shared during educational programs determine the nature of a positive learning in the clinical setting. Judgments need to be made in the practice arena. Judgments should be based on facts and be tempered with human kindness and understanding.

A director of nursing or vice president of nursing should determine his or her philosophy of nursing administration and nursing education. There is evidence that when nursing staff members feel that they have had a voice in the institution's policies they have more positive feelings about their jobs. Blagman (1981) did not, in her research, have the opportunity to review governing structures of hospitals. The need for control of the work environment could be a major factor in her findings. Hard work along with lack of autonomy is a treacherous combination.

It has been observed by the author that risk taking is increased by those nurses who openly express, analyze, and share their personal feelings about professional matters with their colleagues. They thereby have an opportunity to receive constructive feedback from other nurses. This can lead to new perspectives and understanding of their own relationship with patients and colleagues. This process can be greatly enhanced by the institution through the development of support groups, special staff meetings, and social events that help the staff to feel they are understood and appreciated.

Effective feedback about the concern of nurses is another measure to improve decision-making abilities. Organizations that are successful in increasing nursing autonomy have built into their administrative structure procedures for facing up to and resolving job-related frustrations.

Nurses should be occasionally given opportunities to break from stressful situations. This may make the difference between burnout and the development of successful coping mechanisms. The most positive form of a "break" from stressful situations has been called "time out." The nurse during "time out" may voluntarily choose to do some other less stressful type of nursing for a period of time. For example, spending some time each week in a setting where patients are ambulatory and recovering may allow the nurse to see some former patients getting well. Another example is planned times to catch up on the paperwork associated with the job environment.

Nurses need space at work and from work. Whenever one becomes totally absorbed in one activity, other aspects of life are negated. Investment of one's total psychological energy slowly diminishes one's ability to creatively relate to the other aspects of life that bring meaning and fulfillment. A fundamental health principle is that people are happiest when they lead well-balanced lives in which some time and energy is devoted to work, and some to recreation, companionship, and interests other than work.

SUMMARY

Obviously there is not one strategy that can improve decision making. Every human being is different and each copes with decision making somewhat differently. The important message is that each person be in touch with himself or herself and be able to know and recognize when risk taking is appropriate.

Nurses should pay more attention to measures to improve risk-taking behaviors. Nurses should try to understand better those colleagues who lack the capability to take risks. The goal of Blagman's study was to investigate individuals who participate in the decision-making process. To be able to take risks is to be applauded. Blagman views improving the educational process as a way of achieving autonomous decision making. But what are the educational plans for those in administrative positions? Who will prepare risk-taking nursing administrators?

REFERENCE

Blagman, P. Dilemmas in decision making. Unpublished doctoral dissertation, Teachers College, Columbia University, 1981.

[11]

Organized Nurses and Collective Bargaining: Opinions, Participation, and Militance

Elaine E. Beletz

INTRODUCTION

Prior to the 1960s, professionals for the most part were repulsed by the thought of unionism and collective bargaining. The opposition argued in terms of the effects on the profession's status, ethics, public service, and protection of practitioner individualism (Goldenberg, 1968). Researchers found that professionals accepted compatibility between collective bargaining and professionalism as long as collective bargaining did not impinge on professional individuality and strikes were not mentioned (Crispo, 1963; Bairstow, 1974). The increasing acceptability on the part of professionals of the tools of organized labor has undoubtedly been influenced by changing societal values which legitimatize confrontation and the use of collective strength to achieve objectives. Willingness to engage in a strike is no longer antithetic to many professionals' purview. Some researchers are of the opinion that militancy is a pervasive and widely distributed attitude throughout professional groups (Alutto & Belasco, 1974).

The use of collective bargaining by nurses is highly controversial. Emotionalism and misconception prevail. As late as 1976, a nursing ar-

This investigation was partially funded by a research grant from the national organization of Sigma Theta Tau.

ticle advocated the use of personal confrontation as being more acceptable to professionalism than collective bargaining (Hopping, 1976). The
essential attraction of collective group effort is that it provides a means
for the redistribution of power within the employment setting. The ultimate thrust in the adoption of this technique by nurses is the realization of goals directed toward achieving greater power, autonomy, voice,
and control over practice within the work setting. Additional goals include job security, freedom from arbitrary treatment, and elevation of
salaries and benefits to a level of comparability with other salaried professionals in society. However, the mere availability of a collective bargaining program, or even a negotiated contract, is not sufficient to render
collective bargaining viable or effective in achieving one's goals. Integral to the effective use of the process is employee solidarity and participation.

REVIEW OF LITERATURE ON COLLECTIVE BARGAINING

Collective bargaining is an institutionalized power relationship. The relative bargaining power of each of the involved parties may be viewed
as the underlying force behind the labor-management relationship and
the process of agreement (Chamberlain & Kuhn, 1968). The need for
member knowledge and participation emanates from the collective bargaining process. The bargaining agent, the process, and the resultant
agreement strongly impact upon the employee's private as well as professional life. Rosen and Rosen (1955) consider member beliefs a key
to union power as well as a predictor of the degree of support the members are likely to give the bargaining agent. The character of the union
itself was felt to be a conditioning effect on the social and psychological factors that motivate union members to participate in union activities (Tannenbaum & Kahn, 1958). The presence of leaders interested
in taking part in union activities was found to be a necessary ingredient
for motivating workers to participate, even though conditions of dissatisfaction and low morale were present (Sayles & Strauss, 1967).
Though some women have been in the vanguard of the labor movement, for the most part women have been considered difficult to organize and to be "poor" collective bargaining material. Wertheimer and
Nelson (1975) found that women tend to contribute to union activity
as helpers to men; however, women did seem more interested than
men in union affairs.

The research conducted in relation to nurses and collective bargaining has usually addressed itself to attitudes and proclivities toward collective bargaining, participation in work stoppages, attitudes toward

different bargaining agents, and contract preferences. Rarely have the study populations been exclusively limited to nurses organized for collective bargaining purposes.

Miller and Dodson (1976) reviewed the occurrence of job actions among nurses for the years 1960–1974. Demonstrations were the most prevalent form of activity. A greater incidence of demonstrations and mass resignations occurred before 1969 and a higher incidence of strikes were noted after 1969. Growing nurse militancy has defied an occupational norm "that nurses must maintain a dignified demeanor; to march, to demonstrate, or to engage in similar activities have been interchangeably called unprofessional, undignified, and unladylike" (Jacox, 1971, p. 240). Nurses' reluctance to maximize their bargaining power has paralleled other professional groups. However, increasing collective bargaining sophistication, changing norms within professional groups, the impact of the women's liberation movement, and increased professional consciousness has resulted in nurses' increased commitment to the visible demonstration of bargaining power in the labor-management relationship. On the other hand, many nurses have not accepted the concept of the strike; therefore, it is difficult to assess the degree to which attitudinal and behavioral militancy exists among nurses.

Demographic variables affecting nurses' attitudes and perceptions have been identified in several studies. Baird (1968) investigated the attitudes of Ohio nurses toward collective bargaining. No significant differences in attitudes were noted to be associated with marital status, age, occupation of father, labor union membership of father, occupation of spouse, or amount of formal education of spouse. Those respondents who tended to be favorable were nurses whose husbands were members of unions, who were non-Protestant, whose basic nursing education was received in nonhospital programs or who had obtained further education beyond the hospital diploma, who left hospital employment within five years of the study, and who were members of the professional association. Dissatisfaction with salary tends to promote favorable attitudes toward collective bargaining, and older nurses frequently negatively evaluate trade unions and strikes (Meyer, 1970).

In one study, hospital diploma graduates were identified as being the most favorable to the professional association's collective bargaining role and supported their proclivities with greater participation at meetings (Kralewski, 1969). Several studies identified a number of personal statuses which affected participation in a job action. Alutto and Belasco (1974) surveyed nurses and teachers to identify determinants of attitudinal militancy. The nurse-respondents were employed in three hospitals in western New York. Nurses tended to be more favorable to strikes and traditional unions representing professionals. Sex and marital status were not found to be effective discriminators for the variables measured. Younger respondents were more favorable to strikes and unions, whereas those who were older were more favorable to collective bargaining and professional associations.

In general, the research pertaining to nurses and collective bargaining indicates that important attitudinal and participation correlates have been age, religion, membership in the professional nurse association, union membership, and attitude of spouse. Some studies reveal conflicting data relative to positive attitudes toward collective bargaining in relation to Catholicism, advanced education, membership in the professional nurse organization, and older nurses.

THE INVESTIGATION

Participation and perceptions are independent variables which are usually considered reciprocal to one another. Favorable opinions and attitudes toward collective bargaining may lead to greater participation in the process. Participation, on the other hand, has an educational function which can result in a more favorable posture toward the bargaining system in use. As the use of collective bargaining increases in health care, the impact of this formalized and labor relations system on professional nursing practice will need to be identified. It has been suggested that "before accurate predictions can be made regarding action outcomes of professionals and collective bargaining, more work will have to be done on collective bargaining perceptions as they relate to overt behavior" (Sargis, 1977). The paucity of empirical research involving nurses who have adopted collective bargaining indicates that knowledge is sparse and that findings are often in conflict. This investigation, both descriptive and analytical in purpose, was of an exploratory nature relative to organized nurses' opinions and participation in collective bargaining (Beletz, 1979). Specifically, the question addressed was: What are the relationships between perceptions of collective bargaining, participation in collective bargaining, and selected demographic variables among nurses who are employed by voluntary hospitals in New York State who are organized by the New York State Nurses Association for the purposes of collective bargaining?

POPULATION AND SAMPLE

The population selected for this study was registered nurses employed in nonprofit hospitals in the state of New York who were represented for collective bargaining purposes by the New York State Nurses Association (NYSNA). The nonprofit hospital sector was chosen because this particular setting utilizes a pattern of labor relations most akin to traditional industrial relations models established in private industry. The NYSNA is the largest recognized collective bargaining agent for nurses in the United States.

The sample size of 500 was obtained via a computerized systematic sample with random start. The sample represented 5.19 percent of the total universe at the time of data collection. The sampling interval was nineteen.

LIMITATIONS

The findings of this study were limited to New York State registered nurses employed by voluntary hospitals, who were represented by NYSNA. The self-selection process of a mail-back survey limits the findings to being representative of those who had responded to the questionnaire.

DESIGN

The investigation was a descriptive survey utilizing a mail questionnaire. The period of data collection spanned nine weeks and three mailings were distributed. A response rate of 57.8 percent was attained. A total of 13 nurses disqualified themselves for not meeting the criteria for participants in the study. Two hundred sixty-one usable questionnaires were analyzed which accounted for 54.37 percent of the usable sample of 480.

The respondent population was evaluated as comparable to the original sample with respect to type of membership in the professional association, residence, and geographic proportional distribution of nurses who fit the criteria represented by NYSNA throughout the state.

INSTRUMENT DEVELOPMENT

Two major indices were developed. The perceptions of collective bargaining index was a Likert-type scale that probed the intensity of agreement or disagreement to the various items in a range of choices from one to five. An undecided choice was included because of the impact of neutral opinions on collective bargaining, solidarity, support, and power of the bargaining unit and bargaining agent. Six themes were represented among the 30 perception items: (1) general opinions of collective bargaining; (2) opinions relative to nursing and hospital management; (3) the local bargaining unit; (4) pressure tactics; (5) bargaining agent policies; and (6) perceived relative power of the bargaining agent.

Twenty-eight items comprised the self-reporting participation index which was a portion and modification of an index developed by Tannenbaum and Kahn (1958) to measure participation in unions. The index incorporated 15 specific activities and was dichotomous, requiring a yes or no answer. Descriptive questions were included to determine why a particular activity was not engaged in. Additional questions were included with respect to striking and picketing, and demographic questions incorporated 21 major categories of variables. A panel of seven experts was utilized to determine face and content validity. The questionnaire was piloted for reliability and refinement.

TREATMENT OF THE DATA

Reliabilities of the instrument were determined for the survey data and an intercorrelation matrix was used for the creation of a more efficient perception index as well as for the development of four exploratory subindices. Interitem correlations and reliabilities were established for the participation index and an exploratory, dichotomous, self-reporting index of militance. All perception indices were analyzed individually and in relation to respondent participation and militance. Pearson correlations, one-way analysis of variance, and chi square were utilized to identify relationships between the indices. The elaboration model was employed to control for test factors (demographic variables) affecting the relationships. T-tests were employed in analyzing responses of various subsample groups. One-way analysis of variance and chi square were utilized to identify demographic correlates for all of the indices. The acceptable level of significance was established at the 0.05 level.

Three subgroups—officers, supervisors, and nurses who had attained a senior college degree—were created from the sample and were analyzed for differences in mean response among all the indices. Each of the perception items were cross-tabulated with each of the subgroups, participation and militance indices, and each of the participation items.

FINDINGS

Respondents

The respondents were primarily young (19 to 30 years old), Caucasian, Catholic, and graduates of hospital diploma programs. The nurses were atypical in that 39 percent had attained a baccalaureate degree and more than half had supervisory experience, though 71.3 percent were in staff nurse positions at the time of data collection. Most of the respondents had five years of recent uninterrupted practice, reported absolute financial dependence on the income from their positions, worked in 200 to 600 bed hospitals, were from nonunion families, had utilized collective bargaining for less than four years, and had voted in the consent election for a bargaining agent.

Respondents' Opinions

In responding to each of the 30 perception items, the percentage of nurses who were undecided in opinion varied per item, ranging from 5.4 percent to 35.2 percent. Less than 20 percent of the nurses were undecided for 17 opinion items. The prevailing direction of aggregate responses within each of the six themes incorporated in the opinionnaire suggested that:

1. Collective bargaining was viewed as a method of gaining power and control over professional practice and as a mechanism which would provide protection against arbitrary treatment by employers.
2. While advocating the use of the threat of strike at the bargaining table, the respondents did not subscribe to the typical union adage of "no contract, no work." In addition, 65 percent of the nurses indicated that a nurses' strike does impact on nursing's professional image to the public, and 84 percent overwhelmingly agreed that provisions must be made to cover critical care areas during a nurses' strike.
3. Though hospital managements were viewed as uncooperative when disagreements arose in the nurse-employer relationship, they were perceived as preferring nursing's professional association as the collective bargaining representative for nurses.
4. The local bargaining unit is the formal structural unit for nurses who have adopted collective bargaining. The internal affairs of the bargaining unit was perceived to be under membership control, although the bargaining agent was attributed as having control over the determination of demands for negotiation. Bargaining unit officers and delegates were viewed as effective in providing leadership for nurses in the use of collective bargaining; however, they were seen as ineffective in handling nurses' complaints against management.
5. NYSNA was perceived as a powerful bargaining representative; however, the Association's achievements at the bargaining table were viewed as less than comparable to those of other hospital bargaining agents.
6. With respect to the professional association's policies, the respond-

ents were supportive of the multipurpose nature of the organization and were in opposition to an affiliation with organized labor.

PERCEPTIONS OF COLLECTIVE BARGAINING

This major index reflected the overall industrial relations system of the respondents. It contained 22 items. Initially, the distribution was divided into five equal groups, each representing a different type of perception (Table 11.1). The Adversary was considered to be dissatisfied and unsupportive of the collective bargaining framework as measured. Critical nurses were more positive in their opinions; however, they still

Table 11.1 Percentage Distributions for Subdivisions of the Perception Indices

Index	Adversary	Critical	Fence Sitter	Loyalist	Idealist
Perceptions of Collective Bargaining	11	19	32	25	13
Advantages of Collective Bargaining	5	21	33	34	8
Perceived Power of the Bargaining Agent	8	21	26	29	15
Professional Model of Collective Bargaining	9	21	31	29	10
Union Model	8	31	35	18	7

	Con	Neutral	Pro
Perceptions of Collective Bargaining	29	32	39
Advantages of Collective Bargaining	26	33	42
Perceived Power of the Bargaining Agent	29	26	44
Professional Model of Collective Bargaining	30	31	40
Union Model	39	35	26

N=261; Row Totals may not equal 100 due to rounding to nearest whole number tended to be dissatisfied and unsupportive. Fence Sitters did not commit themselves. Loyalists were nurses who were supportive of collective bargaining but would prefer changes to occur in some areas. Idealists were the most enthusiastic and supportive.

The two favorable and two unfavorable groups were collapsed and the distribution was then trichotomized for most of the analysis into "con" (Adversaries and Critical), neutral (Fence Sitters), and "pro" (Loyalists and Idealists) groups. The maintenance of the neutral group was considered essential because of its impact on nurse solidarity and the use of power, and because of its size, comprising nearly one-third of the respondents. In addition, the mean, median, and mode (69.310, 69.750, and 70, respectively) were fairly close to a score of 66 which would have been achieved had the respondents answered undecided to each item.

The aggregate direction of response of the participants indicated favorableness toward their overall collective bargaining system. The indecisiveness of nearly one-third of the respondents was considered characteristic of the controversial nature and transitional state of collective bargaining for nurses which has emerged with the entrance of trade union competition.

Respondents who most positively evaluated their collective bargaining framework were 51 years of age or older, diploma graduates, had graduated during 1954 or earlier, had obtained advanced education, and had attained a bachelor's or master's degree in a nursing major, and resided or worked in the northeast central part of New York State. The least favorable perceptions were noted for nurses age 19 to 30, whose basic nursing education was obtained in an associate degree program, had graduated their nursing programs between 1970 and 1975, had attained bachelor's or master's degrees in non-nursing majors, and lived or worked in the western portion of the state. In addition, t-tests indicated significant differences in mean response between diploma graduates and associate degree/baccalaureate degree graduates.

INVOLVEMENT IN ACTIVITIES OF COLLECTIVE BARGAINING

A rank order placement of the activities queried suggested that respondents were more likely to engage in activities which were passive or required minimal to slightly moderate effort, such as reading the contract and NYSNA literature, voting, and attending meetings. Activities which required visibility, time, and large energy expenditures—for example, assuming elected office or committee work—ranked the lowest (Table 11.2). The respondents were more "local" than "cosmopolitan" in orientations when evaluating involvement in the affairs of the state nursing association as contrasted with the local nursing bargaining unit.

Table 11.2   Rank Order Participation in Activities of Collective Bargaining

Activity	Yes F	Yes %	No F	No %	No Response F	No Response %
1. Familiarity with Contract	201	77.0	58	22.2	2	0.8
2. Read Most Bargaining Agent Literature	200	76.6	59	22.6	2	0.8
3. Voted in Ratification Election	124	47.5	129	49.4	8	3.4
4. Attended Local Bargaining Unit Meetings in the 12 Months Preceding Data Collection	123	47.1	136	52.1	2	0.8
5. Voted Last Local Bargaining Unit Election	117	44.8	143	54.8	1	0.4
6. Bring Up Grievances	102	39.0	142	54.4	17	6.5
7. Voted Last Statewide Professional Association Election	91	34.9	168	64.4	2	0.8
8. Submitted Bargaining Demands	64	24.5	196	75.1	1	0.4
9. Member, Committee Specified in the Contract	30	11.5	231	88.5		
10. Attend Bargaining Agent Conventions	27	10.3	234	89.7		
11. Member, Negotiating Committee	17	6.5	244	93.5		
12. Officer	15	5.7	246	94.3		
13. Delegate	13	5.0	248	95.0		
14. Member, Bargaining Unit Committee	12	4.6	249	95.4		
15. Member, Statewide Professional Association Committee	9	3.4	252	96.6		

N=261

PARTICIPATION IN COLLECTIVE BARGAINING

The participation index incorporated 15 activities such as meeting and convention attendance, assuming elected office, filing grievances, submitting demands for negotiations, and so forth. Approximately three-quarters of the respondents participated in less than 40 percent of the activities queried. The mean, median, and mode fell at approximately 27 percent of the activities. The distribution was initially divided into five equal groups, each reflecting a different degree of participation. The Apathetic (22 percent) participated in only two activities and were considered indifferent and uninvolved in collective bargaining. Card Carriers (51 percent) indicated involvement in three to six activities. The Involved (23 percent) participated in seven to nine activities, and the Committed (2.3 percent) and the Zealous (1.9 percent) were the most active participants in collective bargaining. One respondent reported affirmatively to all 15 activities, and four nurses achieved a score of zero.

The nurses who were most participatory in collective bargaining had worked for five continuous years, had utilized collective bargaining for eight or more years, had voted in the consent election for a bargaining agent, and were employed in a position equivalent to head nurse, supervisor, or clinical specialist.

The distribution was dichotomized for purposes of analysis. The Apathetic and Card Carrier groups were collapsed into one Inactive group (72.8 percent of the nurses) and those who were Involved, Committed, or Zealous were combined into an Active group (27.2 percent). Only 15.7 percent of the respondents reported participation in 50 percent of the activities. It was, therefore, concluded that most nurses organized for collective bargaining do not involve themselves in the process.

RELATIONSHIPS BETWEEN PERCEPTIONS AND PARTICIPATION IN COLLECTIVE BARGAINING

The lack of tradition for collective bargaining and strong role models for professional unionism may result in nurses' development of "invidious" comparisons between the orthodox trade union model and the professional association's model of collective bargaining. In such cases, nurses who actively participate may hold unfavorable opinions toward collective bargaining. It was, therefore, hypothesized that participation in collective bargaining will be inversely related to positive perceptions of collective bargaining.

Nearly 39 percent of the respondents were classified as having positive perceptions of collective bargaining. In addition, the negatively skewed distribution (–0.152) indicated that more respondents' scores were on the positive side of the mean. It was, therefore, concluded that the respondents tended to be positive toward their collective bargaining framework. A nonsignificant, almost negligible, inverse Pearson correlation was obtained between participation and perceptions of collective bargaining. Generally, the literature tends to support a direct relationship between these variables. Since neither the hypothesis nor the generally expected reciprocal relationship between these two variables were supported, it was concluded that among the survey respondents, participation and perceptions of collective bargaining negligibly influence one another.

No significant relationship was identified on cross-tabulation for these variables. Utilizing the elaboration model, a significant inverse relationship was noted when controlling for respondents who indicated "other" as race and had utilized collective bargaining for a half to two years. A large majority of the Active participants for both demographic variables were unfavorable in their perceptions, whereas a greater proportion of Inactives were favorable in their opinions.

Continued exploration with t-tests revealed significant results in terms of mean response. Respondents who were classified as Idealistic in perception tended to be more participatory, and Zealous participators tended to be idealistic in opinion regarding their labor relations framework. On the other hand, the Committed participators were less favorable in their opinions of collective bargaining when contrasted with the Involved participators.

Perception Subindices

The item intercorrelations between the perception items were examined to identify the presence of any subconcepts. Three emerged: Advantages of Collective Bargaining; Perceived Power of the Bargaining Agent; and, Policies of the Association. The items in each of the subconcepts were combined and developed into an index which was statistically analyzed in the same manner as the major perception index of collective bargaining. Reliabilities for each of the indices were determined.

Advantages of Collective Bargaining

This index incorporated four items: collective bargaining provides for greater control over nursing practice; only the professional association can bargain for the professional needs of nurses; collective bargaining prevents management mistreatment; and collective bargaining is the only mechanism for achieving power for nurses within the hospital. The distribution was similar to that of the major index (see Table 11.1). A significant t-test indicated that nurses who zealously participated most favorably perceived the advantages of collective bargaining. A significant relationship between participation and this index was obtained on cross-tabulation for head nurses and respondents who worked part time. Active participants for both demographic variables tended towards favorable opinions, whereas Inactive participants were more neutral in perception.

Perceived Power of the Bargaining Agent

Nine questions encompassed this index. Four pertained to the local bargaining unit and five addressed NYSNA as a bargaining agent. A shift in the distribution of scores was noted (Table 11.1) with respect to a decline in the size of the neutral group from nearly one-third to one-quarter when compared with the other perception indices. In addition, the percentage of respondents comprising the Idealist and "pro" classifications for this index is higher than for any other perception index. Significant differences in mean response were noted for participation between respondents who were "pro" and "con" in opinion of the power of the bargaining agent and between Involved and Committed participators with respect to their opinions of the bargaining agent's power. The data implied that respondents who favorably perceived the power of the bargaining agent were less participatory.

Significant relationships on cross-tabulation were noted between participation and this index for respondents who were Protestant, graduated their basic nursing program between 1960 and 1964, whose immediate family was devoid of union membership, worked in hospitals of 600 beds, and worked the day shift. In all cases, an inverse relationship was observed, whereby a larger proportion of Active respondents negatively perceived the power of the bargaining agent and more Inactive nurses were favorable in opinion.

The Professional Model of Collective Bargaining

An exclusive model of collective bargaining for professionals has not yet been developed. However, it was the investigator's contention that the labor relations system for professionals and blue collar workers differ. One way in which they differ can be found in the policies and ideologies of the bargaining agent. This index refers to NYSNA policies which affect collective bargaining and which are intrinsic to the model of professional unionism utilized by the Association. The policies pertained to strike, picket lines, militancy, nursing administrators, affiliation with organized labor, and the multipurpose philosophy and mission of the organization.

The distribution closely approximated the major perception index (Table 11.1). No significant relationships were identified with participation. On observation, it was noted that more nurses, irrespective of activity level, favorably perceived the professional model of collective bargaining as measured by the policies of the Association.

Among all of the perception indices, this index had the most demographic correlates. Nurses favorable to the professional model of collective bargaining were women, Caucasian, diploma graduates, had graduated in 1954 or before, were head nurses or supervisors, had voted in the consent election, and lived or worked in the northeast central parts of the state. Respondents who tended to be most negative in their opinions were men, Oriental, associate degree graduates, had graduated between 1955 and 1959, were assistant head nurses, and lived or worked in lower Westchester, Bronx, Manhattan, or Staten Island. Nurses who had not voted in the consent election tended to be neutral in opinion. More nurses who were black, Hispanic, and generic baccalaureate graduates tended to negatively evaluate the professional model of collective bargaining.

UNION MODEL OF COLLECTIVE BARGAINING

Though not statistically identified as a subconcept, an exploratory index was created from seven perception items reflecting traditional union philosophies. A definite shift was noted in the distribution of respondents' scores toward a negative evaluation of a union model of collective bargaining (Table 11.1). A significant relationship was obtained between this variable and participation for respondents from the Brooklyn and Long Island region of New York City. Active nurses from this geographic area negatively evaluated the union model, whereas Inactive participators tended to be neutral in their opinions.

In contrast to the opinions of minority groups regarding the professional model of collective bargaining, Oriental nurses were the most favorable to the union model, and black and Hispanic nurses tended to be neutral toward union philosophies. Caucasian nurses were generally nonsupportive of union ideals. A majority of head nurses, supervisors, and clinical specialists negatively evaluated the union model, and staff nurses and assistant head nurses leaned toward neutral perceptions. A larger proportion of diploma and generic baccalaureate graduates negatively perceived the union model and associate degree graduates leaned toward neutral opinions.

Commitment to Militance

The bargaining agent representing the respondents had not relinquished the "no-strike" policy until October 1977, two months prior to data collection. Therefore, respondents had not engaged in either strike or associated picketing activities. Though participation in these activities could not be measured, the ideological commitment to job actions was surveyed because of the importance of these activities to collective bargaining. The respondents were asked if they would walk a picket line if a nurses' strike were called and if they would vote to strike if an impasse were reached on professional or economic issues. An affirmative response was considered an indicator of willingness to be involved and maximize bargaining power in the collective bargaining process.

The descriptive data (see Table 11.3) demonstrated that a majority of the nurses would walk a picket line and vote to strike in the event of impasse over professional issues. The relatively large proportion of nurses who indicated that they would neither engage in picketing nor vote to strike raises questions relative to the effectiveness of such action if a strike were called. Conceptually, one may have difficulty in separating professional issues from their economic costs; however, it does appear that striking for economic reasons was less acceptable to the survey respondents than was striking for professional issues.

A supplementary index entitled Militance was developed to measure respondents' ideological commitment to the use of power in collective bargaining. The index comprised each of the three questions cited ear-

Table 11.3 Respondents and Job Actions

	Yes		No		No Response	
	F	%	F	%	F	%
Walk on a picket line	135	51.7	115	44.1	11	4.2
Strike for economic issues	110	42.1	139	53.3	12	4.6
Strike for professional issues	141	54.0	105	40.2	15	5.7

N = 261

lier. Affirmative answers to any of the questions received a score point value of one. The distribution was "U"-shaped; 98 nurses achieved a score of zero, and 91 a score of three. The distribution was dichotomized into nonmilitant respondents, 129 nurses who had achieved a score of 0-1, and militant respondents, 132 nurses who had attained a score of 2-3.

Significant Pearson correlations (Table 11.4) were obtained for each of the perception indices, participation and militance. Respondents who more actively participated, and favorably perceived the advantages of collective bargaining and the traditional union model were more militant in orientation. Nurses who favorably perceived their collective bargaining framework, and the power of the bargaining agent and the professional model of collective bargaining were nonmilitant. The strongest relationship identified via Pearson correlation was an inverse association (R = -0.49545) between militance and the professional model of collective bargaining. Significant t-tests (Table 11.5) and chi squares (Table 11.6) were obtained for militance and all perception indices other than perceived power of the bargaining agent.

The most important finding of this investigation was that the ideological commitment to the visible use of power significantly impacts on nurses' perceptions of the various facets of their industrial relations system, particularly the professional model of collective bargaining as advanced in the policies of the bargaining agent. It was also noted that militance was frequently associated with demographic variables which demonstrated actively participating respondents holding negative perceptions. Professional organizations are rarely thought of as being militant in orientation. An often-repeated stereotype of nursing organizations is that the leadership comprises little old ladies in tennis shoes who utilize the most genteel and ladylike methods of persuasion which results in an ineffective outcome. The negative opinions of the Active minority, in conjunction with a proclivity toward militance, may be a consequence of a perceived continuing viability of this stereotype.

Demographic Correlates

Two hypotheses were advanced with respect to correlates of the major indices of perceptions and participation in collective bargaining.

1. Participation in collective bargaining will be related to sex, age, education, membership in NYSNA, hospital size, shift worked, full or part-time employment, and supervisory experience.
2. Perceptions of collective bargaining will be related to sex, age, race, religion, number of years as a graduate nurse, years of recent un-

Table 11.4 Pearson Correlations of Militance with each Perception Index and Participation

Index	Correlation	Significance
Union Model	0.37162	0.00001
Advantages of Collective Bargaining	0.21178	0.00057
Participation	0.18294	0.00301
Perceived Power of the Association	−0.13159	0.03360
Perceptions of Collective Bargaining	−0.29424	0.00001
The Professional Model of Collective Bargaining	−0.49545	0.00001

interrupted practice, financial dependence on employment, union membership of a family member, membership in NYSNA, number of years under collective bargaining, hospital size, shift worked, full or part-time employment, education, and supervisory experience.

Of the hypothesized relationships, only position was found to correlate with participation and age, number of years as a graduate nurse, and basic nursing education significantly related to perceptions of collective bargaining. On exploration, other demographic associations were identified for the major indices and subindices. The breakdown within each category has been cited earlier in conjunction with discussion of each of the indices. The significant category of demographic variable for each of the indices was:

Perceptions of collective bargaining was associated with geographic location, basic nursing education, year of graduation from respondent's basic nursing program, and age.

- Advantages of collective bargaining correlated with geographic location, race, and number of years respondents had utilized collective bargaining.
- Perceived power of the bargaining agent associated with geographic location and the year of graduation from the respondent's basic nursing program.
- The professional model of collective bargaining correlated with geogaphic location, basic nursing preparation, year of graduation from basic nursing program, age, race, sex, and position.

Table 11.5 T-Tests Militance and Perception Indices and Participation

Index	Group	N	Mean	Standard Deviation	Standard Error	T-Value	Degrees of Freedom	Signif-icance
Perceptions of Collective Bargaining	Nonmilitant	129	71.9225	8.844	0.779	4.52	259	0.000
	Militant	132	66.7576	9.575	0.833			
Advantages of Collective Bargaining	Nonmilitant	129	13.0155	2.921	0.257	−3.21	259	0.001
	Militant	132	14.1894	2.979	0.259			
Perceived Power of the Association	Nonmilitant	129	26.7674	5.648	0.497	1.72	259	0.088
	Militant	132	25.5758	5.577	0.485			
Professional Model	Nonmilitant	129	32.1395	4.695	0.413	8.61	259	0.000
	Militant	132	26.9924	4.954	0.431			
Union Model	Nonmilitant	129	18.5581	3.836	0.338	−5.86	259	0.000
	Militant	132	21.3561	3.870	0.337			
Participation	Nonmilitant	129	3.9457	2.119	0.187	−2.95	259	0.003
	Militant	132	4.8182	2.629	0.229			

Table 11.6 Cross-tabulations: Militance and Perception Indices and Participation (in percent)

Index	Group	N	Chi Square	Sig	Con	Opinions Neut	Pro
Perceptions of Collective Bargaining	Militant	132	13.33383	0.0013	38.6	31.8	29.5
	Nonmilitant	129			20.2	31.8	48.1
Advantages of Collective Bargaining	Militant	132	6.16708	0.0458	22.7	38.0	49.2
	Nonmilitant	129			28.7	37.2	34.1
Perceived Power of the Association	Militant	132	4.63669	0.0984	34.8	26.5	38.5
	Nonmilitant	129			24.0	25.6	50.4
Professional Model of Bargaining	Militant	132	63.45836	0.0001	47.0	35.6	17.4
	Nonmilitant	129			11.6	25.6	62.8
Union Model	Militant	132	28.39093	0.0001	25.8	36.4	37.9
	Nonmilitant	129			53.5	33.3	13.2
					Inactive		Active
Participation in Collective Bargaining	Militant	132	3.36337	0.0667	67.4		32.6
	Nonmilitant	129			78.3		21.7

- The union model associated with basic nursing preparation, race, and position.
- Participation in collective bargaining correlated with the number of years of recent continuous practice, position, number of years organized for collective bargaining, and having voted in the consent election for a bargaining agent.
- Militance was associated with age, race, religion, basic nursing education, year of graduation from basic nursing program, years of recent continuous practice, membership in the Association prior to collective bargaining, and geographic location.
- No significant correlations were identified for nurses who were financially dependent on the income from their position, union membership of a family member, hospital size, shift worked, or full- or part-time employment status. Those correlates which were significant, particularly seniority, position, age, religion, sex, membership in the Association, involvement in the initial organizing campaign, and geographic location are supportive of previous findings. Since more demographic variables were identified for the professional model of collective bargaining (Table 11.7) and militance (Table 11.8) it would appear that nurses' personal characteristics have a greater impact on perceptions of these two facets of collective bargaining.

Nurses with Senior College Degrees

Nurses who had attained a minimum of a baccalaureate degree in nursing (N=74) were more militant than nonprofessionally educated nurses. It was observed that nurses with a minimum of a senior college degree (N=101), irrespective of major, significantly perceived the Association as less powerful and were more militant than were nurses who had not achieved this credential. More nurses with a minimum of a baccalaureate degree were in favor of a complete strike without provision of coverage for critical care areas or emergencies. They also tended to disagree that the power of registered nurses would improve if the Association represented nonprofessional personnel. Though not significant, it was observed that these nurses had an overall lower participation rate than did the other nurses in the study.

Officers

This subgroup comprised those respondents who had been either an officer, delegate, or member of a negotiating team (N=26; 10 percent of the respondents). No significant differences were detected between

Table 11.7 Cross-tabulations of Demographic Correlates of The Professional Model of Collective Bargaining (in percent)

Variable	N	Chi Square	Significance	Con	Neut	Pro	Group Mean
Sex							
Female	250	4.84318	0.0888*	28.0	30.8	41.2	29.7240
Male	8			62.5	25.0	12.5	25.2500
Race							
Caucasian	156	29.33124	0.0003	20.5	28.2	51.3	30.9744
Black	47			40.4	29.8	29.8	27.8936
Hispanic	8			50.0	37.5	12.5	26.6250
Oriental	20			55.0	30.0	15.0	26.3500
Other	22			40.9	45.5	13.6	27.0000
Basic Nursing Education							
Associate Degree	54	9.31605	0.0537*	38.9	27.8	33.3	28.3148
Baccalaureate Degree	58			39.7	25.9	34.5	28.8448
Diploma	146			21.9	32.9	45.2	30.3014
Year Graduated from basic nursing program							
1976–1977	34	17.53502	0.1306*	32.4	38.2	29.4	28.8529
1970–1975	82			35.4	26.8	37.8	28.9512
1965–1969	40			37.5	20.0	42.5	29.0500

	n						
1960–1964	42			26.2	35.7	38.1	29.4048
1955–1959	22			36.4	31.8	31.8	28.5000
1950–1954	15			13.3	26.7	60.0	33.7333
1949 or before	25			4.0	40.0	56.0	31.7200
Position		20.45929	0.0087				
Staff Nurse	186			30.6	34.4	34.9	29.0538
Asst. Head Nurse	19			52.6	21.1	26.3	27.1053
Specialist/Practitioner	12			33.3	25.0	41.7	29.9167
Head Nurse	32			9.4	25.0	65.6	32.8750
Supervisor	11			27.3	9.1	63.6	31.2727
Voted Consent Election		7.49404	0.0236**				
Yes	137			27.7	24.8	47.4	30.1314
No	117			30.8	37.6	31.6	28.9573
Geographic Location		18.11714	0.0059**				
Western N.Y.S.	15			33.3	33.3	33.3	29.2000
Northeast Central N.Y.S.	41			17.1	24.4	58.5	31.0244
Lower Westchester, Bronx, Manhattan, Staten Island	113			39.8	23.9	36.3	28.8053
Brooklyn, Long Island	88			22.7	42.0	35.2	29.6250

*Statistically significant one-way analysis of variance

**Nonstatistically significant one-way analysis of variance

Table 11.8 Cross-tabulations of Demographic Correlates of An Ideological Commitment to Militance (in percent)

Variable	N	Chi Square	Significance	Nonmilitant	Militant	Group Mean
Age						
19–30	103	24.40342	0.0001	35.9	64.1	1.8155
31–40	82			47.6	52.4	1.5122
41–50	47			63.8	36.2	1.1489
51 plus	26			84.6	15.4	0.5769
Race						
Caucasian	156	8.46428	0.0760*	55.1	44.9	1.3205
Black	47			48.9	51.1	1.5957
Hispanic	8			25.0	75.0	2.2500
Oriental	20			30.0	70.0	2.0500
Other	22			36.4	63.6	1.6364
Religion						
Catholic	130	11.39428	0.0098	41.5	58.5	1.7000
Jewish	13			46.2	53.8	1.7692
Protestant	93			63.4	36.6	1.0860
Other	18			36.4	63.6	1.6667
Basic Nursing Education						
Associate Degree	54	13.62695	0.0011	44.4	55.6	1.6481
Baccalaureate Degree	58			31.0	69.0	2.0000
Diploma	146			58.9	41.1	1.2055

	n	F	p	%	%	Mean
Year of Graduation		33.79612	0.0001			
1976–1977	34			38.2	61.8	1.8235
1970–1975	82			35.4	64.6	1.8171
1965–1969	40			37.5	62.5	1.8000
1960–1964	42			61.9	38.1	1.0952
1955–1959	22			54.5	45.5	1.5455
1950–1954	15			80.0	20.0	0.5333
1949 or before	25			88.0	12.0	0.4800
Years of Recent Continuous Practice		20.79095	0.0003			
One	22			45.5	54.5	1.5909
Two	30			40.0	60.0	1.7667
Three	22			27.3	72.7	2.0000
Four	19			15.8	84.2	2.2105
Five	161			59.6	40.4	1.2298
Membership in the Professional Association Prior to Collective Bargaining		3.72827	0.0535*			
Yes	91			58.2	41.8	1.2527
No	161			44.7	55.3	1.5963
Geographic Location		14.34872	0.0025			
Western N.Y.S.	15			60.0	40.0	1.2667
Northeast Central N.Y.S.	41			56.1	43.9	1.3171
Lower Westchester, Bronx, Manhattan, Staten Island	113			35.4	64.6	1.8053
Brooklyn, Long Island	88			60.2	39.8	1.2273

*Statistically significant one-way analysis of variance

officers and rank-and-file nurses for any of the perception indices or militance. The descriptive data, however, suggested that officers tended to lean more toward a union model of collective bargaining and indicated a lack of involvement in the formalized processes of contract administration.

Supervisors

The supervisory group included respondents who had current or previous experience as a head nurse, supervisor, or nursing administrator. The evidence implied that these nurses were more oriented toward the professional model of collective bargaining, were more participatory in collective bargaining, and were unlikely to endorse either militance or the union model.

SUMMARY

Collective bargaining may be adopted as a means to ameliorate perceived problems in the work environment. The use of this modality by registered nurses has been controversial. Nurses have frequently been characterized as apathetic and submissive and, like other professionals, tend to be uncomfortable with adversarial relationships and techniques of confrontation and militancy. The contemporary nurse, however, may be considered "radicalized" when contrasted to her professional forebears. Increased attitudinal favorability has been noted for both collective bargaining and the use of militant tactics to press demands. This survey was undertaken to describe how nurses who have adopted collective bargaining perceive the various facets of their labor relations system and to identify the degree of involvement in activities associated with collective bargaining. The major findings suggest that:

1. Organized nurses' perceptions of their collective bargaining framework reflect a lack of solidarity and strong opinion-individualism.
2. Organized nurses are nonparticipatory in activities associated with their labor relations framework.
3. Among the survey respondents, perceptions and participation in collective bargaining negligibly influenced one another.
4. Organized nurses' ideological commitment to the visible demonstration of bargaining power strongly impacts on their perceptions and involvement in collective bargaining.
5. Personal status tends to be more closely associated with perceptions of the professional model of collective bargaining and an ideological commitment to militance.

REFERENCES

Alutto, J. A., & Belasco, J. A. Determinants of attitudinal militancy among nurses and teachers. *Industrial and Labor Relations Review*, 1974, *27*, 216–227.

Baird, W. M. *Collective bargaining by registered nurses.* Doctoral dissertation, Ohio State University, 1968.

Bairstow, F. Professionalism and unionism: Are they compatible? *Industrial Engineer*, 1974, *40*, 40–42.

Beletz, E. E. *Collective bargaining and New York State registered nurses in the voluntary hospital sector: Perceptions and participation.* Doctoral dissertation, Columbia University, 1979.

Chamberlain, N. W., & Kuhn, J. *Collective bargaining* (2nd ed.). New York: McGraw-Hill, 1968.

Crispo, J. Collective bargaining and the professional. *Canadian Hospital*, 1963, *40*, 47–49.

Goldenberg, S. B. *Canada task force on labor relations, study #2 professional workers and collective bargaining.* Ottawa: McGill University, 1968.

Hopping, B. Professionalism and unionism: Conflicting ideologies. *Nursing Forum*, 1976, *15*, 372–383.

Jacox, A. Collective action and control of practice by professionals. *Nursing Forum*, 1971, *10*, 239–257.

Kralewski, J. E. *The professional nurse in the hospital organization: A study of conflict resolution.* Doctoral dissertation, University of Iowa, 1969.

Meyer, D. *Determinants of collective action attitudes among hospital nurses: An empirical test of a behavioral model.* Doctoral dissertation, University of Iowa, 1970.

Miller, M. H., & Dodson, L. Work stoppages among nurses. *Journal of Nursing Administration*, 1976, *6*, 41–45.

Rosen, H., & Hudson Rosen, R. A. *The union member speaks.* New York: Prentice-Hall, 1955.

Sargis, N. M. *Collective bargaining in the nursing profession, the hospital "director" as object of special study.* Doctoral dissertation, Columbia University, 1977.

Sayles, L. R., & Strauss, G. *The local union.* New York: Harcourt Brace and World, 1967.

Tannenbaum, A. S., & Kahn, R. L. *Participation in union locals.* New York: Row Peterson, 1958.

Wertheimer, B. M., & Nelson, A. H. *Trade union women: A study of their participation in New York City locals.* New York: Praeger, 1975.

SUGGESTED READINGS

Alutto, J. A. *Correlates of nursing attitudes in a collective bargaining situation.* Master's thesis, University of Illinois, 1965.

Cook, A. H. Dual government in unions: A tool for analysis. *Industrial and Labor Relations Review*, 1962, *15*, 323–349.

Dean, I. R. Social integration attitudes and union activity. *Industrial and Labor Relations Review*, 1954, *8*, 48–58.

Gouldner, H. P. Dimensions of organizational commitment. *Administrative Science Quarterly*, 1960, *4*, 468–487.

Hobart, C. L. *A study of the major influences on nurses collective bargaining at selected Massachusetts hospitals.* Doctoral dissertation, Harvard University, 1971.

Miller, R. L. Development and structure of collective bargaining among registered nurses. *Personnel Journal*, 1971, *50*, 134–140.

Perierra-Mendes, R. H. *The professional union: A study of the social service employees union in the New York City Department of Social Services.* Doctoral dissertation, Columbia University, 1974.

Perline, M. M., & Lorenz, V. R. Factors influencing members participation in trade union activities. *American Journal of Economics and Sociology*, 1970, *29*, 425–438.

Rose, A. M. *Union solidarity.* Minneapolis: University of Minnesota Press, 1952.

Seidman, J., London, J., Karsch, B., & Jagliocozzo. *The worker views his union.* Chicago: University of Chicago Press, 1958.

Simonton, W. E. *Work identification of professional nurses employed in the New York City municipal hospitals.* Doctoral dissertation, Columbia University, 1970.

Spinrad, W. Correlates of trade union participation: A summary of the literature. *American Sociological Review*, 1960, *25*, 237–244.

Response

Rita Reis Wieczorek

Beletz's study in 1979 on organized nurses and collective bargaining was the first in-depth nursing study dealing exclusively with and limited to nurses organized for collective bargaining purposes by a state nurses organization. The study is about power in the labor-management relationship in the health care setting and the process of negotiation to develop a contractual agreement. It involves politics in compromise during contract negotiation periods and in the interpretation of the "life" of a contract. Once a contract is negotiated it becomes the policy in the labor-management relationship.

Beletz studied the perceptions of collective bargaining, the participation in collective bargaining, and selected demographic variables among 261 nurses (Beletz, 1979). A mailed questionnaire was used to collect the data. A 54 percent return rate was obtained. Her study was a descriptive, exploratory one. The research methodology and the analysis of the data is well presented in her report both verbally and in tabular form. The author of this response believes it is a well-done investigation in an area that is one of the most controversial areas in the nursing profession today.

Where do we go from this beginning? A few suggestions are given for direction in the 1980s.

1. This study should be repeated in other states similar to and dissimilar to New York state. The findings could then be generalized to a larger population, and questions concerning the uniqueness of New York state in reference to collective bargaining could be proven or laid to rest.

2. The climate in the nursing profession toward the perception and/ or participation in the collective bargaining process is everchanging. While the respondent does not question the findings of Beletz's study in 1979, what about the 1980s? Some researchable questions are related to the concept of unionism in general for health professionals and society's reaction to nurses and the health care industry now—and in the future.

3. Contractual gains were made in salary, benefits, and the working environment in the late 1970s and early 1980s. With rising health care costs and governmental regulation, one may ask, who can afford all those nurses in the acute care setting? Have experienced nurses priced themselves out of the marketplace?

4. What is going to happen to collective bargaining during and after implementation of the diagnostic related groups (DRGs)? What staff mix for the acute care setting is most cost-effective?

5. The issue of nurses being represented by professional State Nurses Associations versus "trade" unions has really never been settled. In nursing, one can find the whole gamut of opinion from professional to trade to no union at all.

6. Nationally, unionism is strong. Supposedly, one out of five workers in this country belongs to a union (Bureau of National Affairs, 1983). Trade unions are preparing to make large-scale organizing attempts in some geographical areas. The 1199 union is planning such an approach in the midwest (Bureau of National Affairs, 1983). Can a trade union represent individual professional nurses in the work arena? Are they interested in standards of care and quality assurance?

7. In 1982–1983, the National Labor Relations Board has had approximately 20 plus cases that involve attempts to decertify State Nurses' Associations from representing nursing units for collective bargaining purposes. Can professional associations withstand these challenges?

8. The National Labor Relations Board (NLRB) has, in 1983, several cases that relate to a challenge of having an all-registered nurse (RN) bargaining unit. It has been in the past a practice of the NLRB to support the rights of all RN units. What happens to nursing if the NLRB reverses this decision? This may mean that nurses could be placed in unions with other health professionals. Could a State Nurses' Association represent other health professionals?

9. What affect does unionism have on the practice of nursing? This question has not really been addressed in research. There are states in which nurses are highly organized by State Nurses' Associations, yet there are some areas in which nurses are not organized for collective bargaining purposes in any significant numbers.

10. The tenth and last point to consider is how do collective bargaining perceptions relate to the overt behavior of nurses (Sargis, 1977)? Certainly nurses interested in labor relations would agree that more research is needed in this area.

The reader is asked to return to Beletz's (1984) research in Part II. The investigation deserves to be studied more than once. Beletz has made a giant step forward in removing emotionalism and misconceptions from her investigation. Unfortunately, this is only one study by one person. In honesty, the respondent would be remiss if the statement was not made that emotionalism and misconceptions are still associated with the use of collective bargaining by nurses.

REFERENCES

Beletz, E. *Collective bargaining and New York State registered nurses in the voluntary hospital sector: Perceptions and participation.* Doctoral dissertation, Columbia University, 1979.

Beletz, E. Organized nurses and collective bargaining: Opinions, participation, and militance. In R. R. Wieczorek (Ed.), *Power, Politics, and Policy in Nursing.* New York: Springer Publishing Company, 1984.

Bureau of National Affairs, White Collar Report, National Hospital Union Nurses "Blueprint for Action," Vol. 54, 11:16, 1983, pp. 455–458.

Sargis, N. Collective bargaining in the nursing profession: The hospital "director" as object of special study. Doctoral Dissertation, Teachers College, Columbia University, 1977.

INDEX

Index